Medical Decisions in the face of Uncertainty (Revised)

Jerome Malitz

Seth Malitz

Copyright © 2018 Jerome Malitz & Seth Malitz
Cover by Jerome Malitz & Seth Malitz

All rights reserved.

ISBN: 1729536689
ISBN-13: 978-1729536681

DEDICATION

To wife and mom, Susan, for her unwavering patience, good cheer, and warm dinners, while the writing of this book went on and on.

Contents

Preface 3
Ch. 1: What's It all about? 9
Ch. 2 Best Healthcare in the World? 19
   Regional variation in the rate of surgical procedures 21
   Some of the drivers of over-treatment 24
   Hospitals – putting the patient at risk 25
   Variation in the pricing of medical services 25
   The FDA – not the guardian you think 26
   So where does this leave us? 27
Ch. 3 Static Thinking in Dynamic Times 29
   Conversation with a mathematician and computer scientist 31
   Conversation with another mathematician and computer scientist . 33
   Conversation with a veterinarian 34
   Conversation with Joe and Jane patient 34
   Conversation with a head-and-neck surgeon 35
   Conversation with an internist 36
   Conversation with a pediatric surgeon 37
   Visit to the dermatologist 38
   Conversation with a plastic surgeon 39
   The way doctors (shouldn't) think 40
   Battling the old guard 44
Ch. 4 Winners and Losers 47
   Patients among the winners and losers 48

Doctors among the winners and losers 48

The poor will be winners 49

Abuses by the legal drug lords 51

Chalk one up for the opioid cartel 54

Off-label drug use 56

Unregulated use of laboratory developed tests 57

Regulation of surgery and devices 58

Boost to your health with dietary supplements? 62

Recreational drug use 64

Ch. 5 The Future Starts Today 65

That I should lose to this idiot! 66

Mapping the inner you 69

Game On! 70

Too exciting not to mention 71

A revolution in medical thinking 73

Ch. 6 Medical Decisions in the Face of Uncertainty 75

By the numbers 76

Slow down 77

Ch. 7 What are the Odds? 81

The probabilistic view can be your friend 82

Probability by counting 83

Probability when outcomes are not equally likely 89

Probability on infinite populations 90

Probability histograms 94

Other bar charts 96

Over-binning 98

What exactly is probability? 99

Ch. 8 Conditional Probability and Bayes' Formula 103

Conditional probability 106

Conditional probability and the anti-vax activists 108

Independent events 109

The ideal sample 110

The elusive gold standard 111

Bayes' Theorem 113

Ch. 9 The Right Sample Size 117

The average and other measures of central tendency 118

Variance and standard deviation 122

Mean and variance for distribution curves 124

Mean and variance in higher dimensions 125

The Binomial distribution 126

Probability concentration about the mean 128

Sample size to estimate a population mean 132

Confidence interval explained in a nutshell 136

Confidence interval from sample size and mean 137

Statistical hypothesis testing 137

Estimating things besides a population mean 140

Watson guarding the old guard 140

Combining data 145

Bias and bias compounded 148

Simpson's Paradox 149

Subdividing data 151

Data dredging (fishing, snooping, mining) 152

Cherry-picking by Big Pharma 155

Ch. 10 Progress by Regression 157

The model is the message 159

Getting the "best" fit from a family of models 163

Getting the "right" family of models 166

Fitting to a bar chart 168

Sometimes there is no good predictive model 170

The most important factors 171

Interpolation and extrapolation 173

Curves as data points 175

Getting the best cutoff value 177

Getting the best cutoff boundary 179

Ch. 11 Decisions, Decisions, Decisions 183

Is it safe? Is it effective? 184

ARR, RRR, and NNT 186

Histograms of benefits and harms 189

Were you satisfied with your treatment? 192

Decision trees 193

Hip implant surgery 196

Leaning on the decision tree 202

The Angelina Jolie story 203

The Angelina Jolie story (continued) 204

Aching back 206

Prostate cancer 207

In a heartbeat 209

The Rolling Stones put it this way 210

Ch. 12: *79.48% of statistics are made up on the spot* 215

"Statistics" leading us astray 216

The medium is the message 224

From casino to clinic 229

Why isn't rigorous statistics used more in medicine? 231

So where should you put your trust? 233

Ch. 13 Nothing but the Best 235

But I'm special 237

In the public interest 238

Alternative medicine 239

Evidence-based medicine in Botswana 241

Conflicted medical practice 242

Blunders in Western medicine 245

Hope and desperation 248

Comparing medical traditions 249

If it works, it works 251

A revolution in the way medical decisions are made 254

Where's the Bibliography? 259

Index 261

ACKNOWLEDGMENTS

Our thanks and gratitude to the following people for helpful conversations that influenced the writing of this book:

E. Lee Nelson, MD, neurosurgeon
Sameer Oza, MD, cardiologist
Satish Rao, MD, neurologist
George Russell, MD, dermatologist
Lynn Voss, MD, orthopedic surgeon

And the team at Spine West, Boulder:
Cliff Gronseth, MD, physical medicine & rehabilitation
Vaheed Sevvom, PA-C, physical medicine & rehabilitation
John Toby, MD, physical medicine & rehabilitation

Thanks to our long-time colleague Prof. Richard Holley for answering some technical questions.

Thanks to Eliza Cross, Denise Davis - PT, and Tony Dudek.

Thanks to son and brother, Jed, for his invaluable comments.

And many thanks to wife and mom, Susan, who helped with proofreading and made many helpful suggestions.

Preface

Healthcare in the US is a mess: quality is wanting and cost is out of control. Nearly one out of every five dollars earned is spent on healthcare, and the number keeps climbing. Our per-capita outlay in this realm is far greater than that of any other industrialized nation, and yet we have worse patient outcomes to show for it. This in spite of the fact that U.S. medical research remains the primary global source for new discoveries, drugs, medical devices, and clinical procedures. The US system is rife with over-treatment, ineffective and harmful treatment, and unnecessary medical tests. Many of our citizens get shoddy care or no care at all.

The problem is not new. We've been talking about it for years: "We need to reform the system. We need a new paradigm for health care. We need more transparency. We need medical care that has better justification. We need *true evidence-based medicine*." It all seems so obvious. But what exactly do we mean by "true evidence-based medicine"? How do we get it?

True evidence-based medicine is the product of *rigorous statistics*, a data-gathering and -analysis methodology built on incontrovertible mathematics. Not only can it estimate the likelihood that a treatment will work for you, but it can offer a meaningful guarantee on the reliability of that estimate. This kind of information enables you to compare treatment options in an objective, quantitative way, so as to help you make the best treatment decision. It's the kind of information you ignore at your peril. And you don't want to ignore it in other realms either, such as when buying a car, a home, a major appliance, an investment, an education, health insurance, or placing a bet on your favorite sport's team.

Rigorous statistics provides an objective, unbiased way of understanding the world, and reports its results in a transparent manner: The audience knows how the numbers were arrived at and how reliable they are. It's a far cry from the numbers typically thrown at us in the media in a brazen effort to sell stuff or distort opinion, thrown at us without explaining their origin and without any guarantee of reliability. It's that kind of stuff that we call *flimflam stats*. Making a medical decision based on flimflam stats is reckless, if not utterly foolish.

However, it takes a little while to explain what *rigorous statistics* is. It requires that we know something about the mathematical concept of probability and its logical consequences. That such a branch of mathematics exists may seem strange to some, since math is thought to be all about certainty, while probability is all about chance. Yet it does exist, and through it we have come to understand the world with greater clarity and greater depth than ever before.

This book explains the basic underpinnings of *rigorous statistics*, and will leave the reader with no doubt that it's backed by rock-solid, irrefutable mathematics, and not just the wild hype of a couple of over-zealous mathematicians. We don't want the reader to accept any material just on our say-so.

Rigorous statistics has been around for a long time, and has been used extensively in fields outside medicine. But it hasn't been adopted as the primary guide for making medical decisions on a daily basis. That's mainly because doctors have not been trained in statistics. But also because, until recently, the requisite computer systems and necessary stores of standardized historical patient data have not been available to make true patient-centric, clinical care a reality.

But now the requisite computer capabilities are here and so is much standardized historical patient data – not for all medical conditions and not for all patient types, but enough to be of great value to many patients and the healthcare system in general. In time, as more patient data arrives, the range of applications will increase, covering more conditions and more kinds of patients. We are poised for a new age in clinical practice, in which patient-centric, *rigorous statistics* are used as the primary advice for medical decisions. Compared to the archaic way medical decisions are made today, the new paradigm well-deserves to be called *revolutionary*.

As in all revolutions, there will be winners and losers: Big Pharma, device manufacturers, mega-hospitals, and certain doctors will have their share of losers. Patients will be on the winning side.

This book is for patients, healthcare professionals, and healthcare policymakers, as well as journalists who report on medical issues. It's for anyone interested in delivering or receiving better and more affordable health care.

Jerome Malitz & Seth Malitz

JEROME & SETH MALITZ

Part I

Today's Healthcare – In Dire Need of a Revolution

JEROME & SETH MALITZ

Ch. 1: What's It all about?

To paraphrase the oft-paraphrased master of rhetoric, Aristotle: *First we'll tell you what we're going to tell you; then we'll tell you; then we'll tell you what we told you. And that's what we'll do.* So here we begin with a chapter by chapter synopsis of the book; then we'll present the chapters; then we'll do a bit of a recap. The book has three parts:

Part I
Today's Healthcare – In Dire Need of a Revolution

The per capita cost of US healthcare is by far the highest in the world, yet the quality of US healthcare is well below that of other nations according to various outcome metrics.

Much of this is due to poor decision-making by the medical profession, where doctors generally select treatment based on med-school training, limited personal experience, intuition, heuristics, hearsay, habit, and sometimes business considerations. Too often that choice is not the one that will best serve the patient. It's an antiquated paradigm that ignores the role computers, statistical analysis, and historical patient data could be playing. Compared to other fields, the medical profession has been slow to enter the Information Age, where data is assiduously gathered, digitized, archived, and statistically analyzed by computer, to form a rigorous, evidential basis for good decisions and actions.

It's this approach that's so desperately needed in medical decision-making, where the paradigm shift could rightly be called revolutionary.

Ch.1: What's It All About?

Here's where you are right now.

Ch. 2: Best Healthcare in the World?

Does the US have the best healthcare system in the world? Hardly! A litany of evidence points to a glut of poor health outcomes and ruinous financial cost. The system is rife with overtreatment, ineffective and harmful treatment, and unnecessary medical tests. This stems primarily from poor decision-making by the medical profession. But as we will see, there are ways to confront the problem.

Ch. 3: Static Thinking in Dynamic Times

Science and technology are increasingly reshaping every aspect of our lives, including medical practice.

But the decision-making component of medical practice remains stuck in the past. It doesn't have to be that way. Today, we have the means to deliver rigorous, personalized, evidence-based medicine. The requisite ingredients are all there: computing power, statistical methodology and algorithms, and large volumes of historical patient data in the form of electronic medical records that are becoming increasingly standardized.

Yet the medical profession is reluctant to admit the benefits of this approach, reluctant to admit that a computer can deliver better information, better advice, and often better decisions than a doctor. We beg to differ.

Ch. 4: Winners and Losers

The rigorous statistical approach to medical decision-making based on computerized analysis of standardized electronic medical records is different enough from the way medical decisions are made today that it can rightly be called revolutionary. The goal of the revolution is to use math, statistics, computers, and data to remove as much subjectivity and corrupting influence as possible from medical decision-making. The only subjectivity that should be allowed to enter into a treatment decision is that of the patient expressing his own personal goals.

In this revolution, as with every revolution, there will be winners and losers.

One group of losers will be drug manufacturers and distributors who engage in direct-to-consumer advertising; set prices inconsistent with drug performance; make fraudulent claims for efficacy, safety, and side effects; don't recall dangerous drugs in a timely manner; and benefit from unwarranted off-label drug prescriptions. Another group of losers will be device manufacturers whose products are poorly regulated, and who often drag their feet in recalling hazardous items. Other losers will be hospital directors who pressure doctors to perform tests and procedures to feed the bottom-line. Doctors who push unwarranted tests and procedures of their own volition will also be losers. Laboratories that manufacture and market diagnostic tests of poor quality will be losers. Makers and distributors of dietary supplements who promote their wares based on unsubstantiated claims of efficacy and safety will be losers, as will be the larger alternative medicine industry, for similar reasons.

Among the winners will be patients who want personalized, reliable, evidence-based information on treatment performance. People all over the world will benefit from the revolution – even those in the poorest countries and rural areas, assuming they have access to health care staff who are instructed in best-practice care or who can access telemedicine or the Internet.

Ch. 5: The Future Starts Today

Though the medical profession and some patients balk at the idea that computers can deliver better advice and often better decisions than a doctor, that perspective is increasingly at odds with what current technology tells us is possible.

Today, in all sorts of ways, we are reaping the fruits of fast computer hardware, massive on-chip memory, prodigious data storage, and high-speed computer networks. We see the significant role that computers and robots already play in manufacturing and quality control. We now have cars and trucks that are able to drive themselves. Numerous smart apps are available for our smart phones. Computers in the financial sector do real-time market analysis and stock trading. Computers can beat the best human players in chess and other games of strategy. Astonishing milestones have been attained recently in machine learning, computer vision, natural language processing, and autonomous robot-motion control.

We recognize how capable computers are in realms outside medicine – shouldn't we be using them more inside medicine?

Ch. 6: Medical Decisions in the Face of Uncertainty

Uncertainty has always been part of life, and it's always been a challenge to find ways to cope with it.

The mathematics of probability and statistics tells us how confidently we can infer or estimate something about the world from empirical observations. It has provided astonishing insights into the way the world works, and has played a major role in advancing science, engineering, and medicine.

But in medical decision-making, we have barely tapped into this paradigm. Yet it's the only paradigm that gives meaning to the words "rigorous, evidence-based medicine".

Part II
In the Face of Uncertainty

When decisions have to be made in the face of uncertain outcomes, it's helpful to know the odds of those outcomes, the probabilities. In some cases, those probabilities can be known exactly, as with games at the casino. But most of the time they have to be estimated from experimental observations or by sampling from populations of individuals. When probabilities have to be estimated, it's important to know the reliability of those estimates. Toss a coin a hundred times and observe the fraction of heads – how well does that number estimate the intrinsic bias of the coin? This kind of question, and many like it of medical significance, are answered by the mathematics that underlies *rigorous statistics*. Understanding the main concepts of rigorous statistics is crucial for many applications, and in particular, for the pursuit of evidence-based medicine. Fortunately, you don't have to be a mathematician or statistician to grasp the basics.

Ch. 7: What Are the Odds?

Whether placing a bet on the big game or a medical procedure, we want to know the odds – the probability of a particular outcome. And often we'll make an important decision based on that probability.

But what is probability? How is it calculated? Most people don't realize it, but there is actually a mathematical theory with all the usual precision, rigor, and certainty that we expect from mathematics, that deals with chance. It is one of the greatest achievements in all of science. Our aim in this chapter is to introduce the reader to the basic concepts of probability theory, explain how and why it works, and illustrate the ideas with examples.

Ch. 8: Conditional Probability and Bayes' Formula

Many important practical questions are of the form: "What is the probability that event A will happen given that event B has occurred?" Or more succinctly: "What is the probability of A given B?" This is a question about *conditional probability*. Simple as it might sound, people often get tripped up by it, and make poor medical decisions as a result. The anti-vaccination crowd is a prime example, mixing up their A's and B's, with negative consequences.

Bayes' Formula is an important mathematical relationship between conditional probabilities, widely used in practice, that sometimes leads to unexpected conclusions.

Ch. 9: The Right Sample Size

Questions such as, "What fraction of the population who took medication M avoided harmful event H?", often involve populations so large or so difficult to canvas that trying to do so is impossible. So we try to estimate the answer by looking at an unbiased sample from the population. But how large a sample is required in order to be "acceptably confident" that the rate at which H occurs in the sample is a "good" approximation to the rate at H occurs in the population? The required sample size is often far smaller than you might think – and this is what makes a great deal of scientific research, particularly in medicine, practical. Mathematics tells us the sample size necessary to achieve any desired degree of reliability in the sample estimate.

Meta-analysis is a popular research paradigm these days in which a number of existing statistical studies are combined into a single study. This activity, which is distinct from producing a survey article, is rife with pitfalls, and often amounts to an abuse of statistics in that there is no meaningful measure of reliability on the results.

Ch. 10: Progress By Regression

Regression analysis is math-speak for a disciplined way of fitting curves and surfaces to data points in two, three, and higher dimensions, "smoothing" the data and highlighting the essential trend that relates an output measurement to one or more input measurements. The data points might correspond to readings from different patients, or readings from a single patient over time.

A fitted curve can illustrate how diastolic blood pressure varies with systolic blood pressure, or how max heart rate varies with age. A fitted surface can illustrate how risk of heart attack varies with waist-to-hip ratio and cholesterol level. If the data points are from a single patient over time, then a curve fit can show the time-dependent trend of those readings. This may be of diagnostic and treatment value.

A curve fit of data points can itself be represented as a data point, and this can be useful in deciding whether a patient's measurement trend calls for an intervention.

Regression analysis is concerned not only with fitting curves and surfaces to data points, but also with the quality and reliability of the fit. It addresses questions like: What kind of curve or surface should be used for the fit? How tight is the fit? How large a sample is necessary to be "acceptably confident" that the fit to the sample is a "good" estimate of the fit to the population?

When many types of input measurements are available, regression analysis can identify those that are most useful in predicting the output measurement. If there is a causal relationship between these particular input measurements and the output measurement, then controlling the former can be used to control the latter – knowledge that can be of great medical benefit.

Ch. 11: Decisions, Decisions, Decisions

A treatment that might benefit the patient in some ways, can potentially harm the patient in others. When deciding among treatments, it's useful to compare them based on the odds of being helped, the odds of being harmed, and numerical guarantees as to how well these odds are known. This information can be obtained from rigorous statistics on samples of historical patients like the current patient. The results can be expressed in easy-to-understand ways that can serve as patient decision aids.

One group of decision aids consists of numbers with acronyms like ARR (absolute risk reduction) and RRR (relative risk reduction), which are measures of a treatment's potential to benefit, and ARI (absolute risk increase) and RRI (relative risk increase), which are measures of a treatment's potential to harm. Each of these numbers is estimated from a comparison of two samples of historical patients, one sample that received the treatment and one that didn't. Knowing a treatment's ARR is often more useful than knowing its RRR. Yet many drugs are marketed by RRR because it's a bigger, more impressive-sounding number, and hence better for sales, but it does not convey how likely it is that you will be helped by the drug.

Often it makes more sense to ask, "What level of benefit (or harm) might I get from this treatment?", rather than, "Could this treatment benefit (or harm) me?" Here, a useful decision aid is a benefit (or harm) histogram built from a sample of historical patients, showing the fraction of patients who experienced each level of benefit (harm).

Another decision aid is a tree-like diagram called a *decision tree*. It captures the idea that a treatment option often does not have a guaranteed result, and so will lead to one of several chance outcomes, which may then lead to other treatment decisions later, and so on. Taken as a whole, the tree captures the various medical trajectories that the patient might follow. Ideally, the chance branches are labeled with their probability of traversal as estimated from a sample of historical patients.

Decision aids like those above can help the patient make a reasoned decision about which treatment to go with. Not always is there a clear-cut winner, but the aids serve to highlight which treatments are most likely to satisfy the patient's goals.

Part III
Towards Rigorous, Personalized, Evidence-based Medicine

US healthcare is rife with over-treatment, ineffective and harmful treatment, and unnecessary medical tests. Patients are usually ill-equipped to play a role in treatment selection and typically rely on the doctor to make the choice for them. But too often, the resulting treatment decision lacks good evidential support and does not best serve the interests of the patient.

We need a revolution in the way medical decisions are made, a revolution that will bring about rigorous, personalized, evidence-based medicine. Such revolution is ready to go forward, but it depends crucially on understanding the difference between *rigorous statistics* and what we call *flimflam stats*. The former comes with a meaningful guarantee as to how well treatment performance on a sample predicts treatment performance on the larger population. The latter does not. The confusion between rigorous statistics and flimflam stats has been an obstacle to the realization of rigorous, evidence-based medicine. Only by overcoming this confusion can the revolution proceed.

Ch. 12: *79.48% of all statistics are made up on the spot*
Attribution????

We are awash in statistics, often not obtained or reported honestly or competently. We distinguish between two kinds of statistics: *rigorous statistics* and *flimflam stats*.

Rigorous statistics involves collecting an unbiased sample from the target population and using rock-solid mathematics to quantify how "confident' we are that what we observe in the sample is a "good" approximation to what we would observe in the population. This mathematical guarantee of reliability is universally understood and accepted.

By contrast, flimflam stats do not come with any credible measure of reliability. Flimflam stats are typical of numbers thrown at us by the media, numbers designed to sell stuff and persuade, not to convey truths and inform. Trust these numbers at your peril.

Ch. 13: Nothing But the Best

Nothing but the best – of course, that's what we all want, especially if it concerns our health. We want the best drugs, the best treatments, and the best outcomes, all at affordable cost. But that's not what we're getting with US healthcare. We need a revolution, a revolution in how medical decisions are made.

Doctors and patients need to understand what is meant by "rigorous, evidence-based, medical practice", and that this kind of care is what best serves the patient. Doctors and patients need to take full advantage of the available technology – computers, standardized electronic medical records, and rigorous statistics – to ensure that this kind of care gets delivered.

Here's to the revolution!

Ch. 2 Best Healthcare in the World?

The optimist believes this is the best of all possible worlds; the pessimist fears it is true.

James Branch Cabell

One thing for sure, believing that this is as good as it gets quashes the search for something better. But looking for something better than the best doesn't make sense either.

Best healthcare system in the world! That's what US politicians said in 2012, and it's still believed by many in the public today. But not everyone agrees.

According to the World Health Organization's (WHO) 2000 report, the United States spent more per capita on healthcare than any country in the world and yet ranked 37th among 191 nations based on a combined measurement of overall population health, responsiveness of the healthcare system, level of service depending on a person's economic status, and fairness in the distribution of the financial burden. Though the study is often-cited, there is a degree of controversy revolving around the measures used in the analysis and the assumptions made when certain types of data were lacking. A more conservative analysis in the same report put the US at 15th. (See the article, "John Boehner says U.S. healthcare system is best in world", July 5, 2012, on politifact.com.) Others dismiss the findings as simply reflecting poor lifestyle choices by the US population and a lack of universal health coverage, and not reflective of the quality of care itself.

Avoiding some of the criticisms of the WHO study, the Commonwealth Fund's 2004 report, *Mirror, Mirror* of eleven modern industrialized nations – Australia, Canada, France, Germany, the Netherlands, New Zealand, Norway, Sweden, Switzerland, the United Kingdom, and the United States – still ranked the US last on measures of health outcomes, access, efficiency, and equity. That low ranking has persisted through all the subsequent *Mirror, Mirror* reports, issued in years 2006, 2007, 2010, 2014, and 2017. (Google "Mirror, Mirror 2017: International Comparison Reflects Flaws and Opportunities for Better U.S. Health Care".)

Today, the per capita cost of healthcare in the US is two to three times higher than that of nearly all the other countries in the *Mirror, Mirror* reports. (Google "Peterson Foundation 2016 Per Capita Healthcare Costs International Comparison".) Total healthcare spending in the US represents 18% of GDP, and is expected to rise to 20% by year 2025. The federal government is the largest payer of these healthcare expenditures, which cover Medicare, Medicaid, and subsidized health insurance.

A 2010 article in *The New England Journal of Medicine*, "Ranking 37th – Measuring the Performance of the US Health Care System", makes the point that even if the 2000 WHO study has its critics, the following are not in dispute: the United States in 2006 was number one in terms of healthcare spending per capita, but ranked 39th for infant mortality, 43rd for adult female mortality, 42nd for adult male mortality, and 36th for life expectancy. (For more recent health outcome rankings Google "Peterson Foundation 2016 International Ranking Health Outcomes".)

The disconnect in the US between per capita cost of healthcare and access to healthcare is shameful. But it's the *quality* of the health care being delivered, especially in relation to its cost, that is our concern here – the high levels of over-treatment, ineffective and harmful treatment, and unnecessary medical tests. This state of affairs reflects a lack of standards in medical practice and a failure by the medical community to adopt a more rigorous, evidence-based approach to medical decision-making. Patients, meanwhile, lack adequate information about the risks and benefits of treatment options, and in the belief that doctors know best, delegate the decision-making to their physicians.

Regional variation in the rate of surgical procedures

According to the well-known Dartmouth Atlas of Healthcare (assembled by The Dartmouth Institute for Health Policy and Clinical Practice), in New England between 2007 and 2010, the number of tonsillectomies performed annually on children ranged from 2.7 per 1000 kids in Bangor, Maine to 10.9 per 1000 kids in Littleton, New Hampshire – a four-fold variation. Tonsillectomy is used most often for obstructive sleep apnea and recurrent throat infections. However, the Dartmouth researchers strongly question its usefulness except in cases of severe recurrent infection. The researchers state that few high-quality studies support the practice in general.

Today, roughly 600,000 hysterectomies are performed in the US each year. The national rate dropped by 36% from 2002 to 2010, and has since stabilized, but there is still a disturbing amount of regional variation in the use of the procedure. (See p. 4 of the book, *Hysterectomy: Exploring Your Options, second edition*, 2015.) Hysterectomy rates also vary widely across Western countries. The rates go from a high of 5.4 per 1000 women in the US to a low of 1.2 per 1000 women in Norway. (See the article "Overview of current trends in hysterectomy", *Expert Rev of Obstet Gynecol*, 2009.) The annual healthcare cost of hysterectomies in the US is over $5 billion.

Today, about 1.3 million newborns are delivered by Cesarean section (C-section) in the US each year. From 1996 to 2007, the rate rose by 53% and now represents about a third of all US births. A 2015 article, "C-Sections increase risks for mothers and infants" by the Consumer Reports Health Ratings Center, describes a 2009-2012 study on the variation in C-section rates across hospitals in the US. The study found extreme variation, and questions whether the procedure is being grossly overused on women who would otherwise have low-risk births. For example, the C-section rate at one Los Angeles hospital was 55% while at another it was only 15%. Such discrepancy is repeated throughout the nation. Some hospitals have C-section rates ten times higher than others. The annual healthcare cost of C-sections in the US is over $10 billion.

The Consumer Reports article states that healthy, low-risk women who undergo a first C-section are three times more likely to suffer serious complications compared with natural birth. The risk increases with each use of the procedure. Furthermore, C-section takes longer to recover from than vaginal delivery and often leads to prolonged pain.

The Dartmouth Atlas of Health Care webpages on "Variations in Surgical Procedures" (see variation_surgery_2 and variation_surgery_3) refer to their study from 2008 to 2010, which found striking regional variation in the rates of other common surgeries including: back surgery; hip and knee replacement; gallbladder removal; radical prostatectomy; coronary artery bypass; lower extremity bypass; carotid endarterectomy; and percutaneous coronary intervention. (For other detailed information, see the Dartmouth Atlas reports in the 2014 series, "Variation in the Care of Surgical Conditions". See also the article "Understanding regional variation in the use of surgery", *Lancet*, Sept. 28, 2013, and available on the website ncbi.nlm.nih.gov.)

According to the Dartmouth Atlas of Health Care webpage with title "Preference-Sensitive Care" (link dartmouthatlas.org + /keyissues/issue.aspx?con=2938) and the associated topic brief (dartmouthatlas.org/downloads/reports/preference_sensitive.pdf), there are two principal causes of such extreme regional variation (quotes in italics):

First, there is the often poor state of clinical science; for many conditions for which major surgery is an option, the [different possible] treatments have not been adequately evaluated through rigorous [statistical] studies. Thus, when surgeons recommend surgery, they often do so on the basis of subjective opinion, personal experience, anecdote, or an untested clinical theory...

Second, patients commonly delegate decision-making to physicians, under the assumption that doctors can accurately understand patients' values and recommend the correct treatment for them. Yet studies show that when patients are fully informed about their options [the risks and benefits, and the likelihood of each] they often choose very differently from their physicians.

[The observed variation] suggests that local medical opinion has a strong influence on choice of treatment.

The Dartmouth researchers advocate for patients being more involved in treatment selection. They recommend that patients be provided with decision aids that communicate *high-quality, up-to-date information about the condition, including risks and benefits of available [treatment] options and, discussion of the limits of scientific knowledge about outcomes.*

Characterizing what is meant by "high-quality information" and "limits of scientific knowledge about outcomes" is a major thrust of this book.

In the Dartmouth Atlas webpages titled "FAQ" (at the link dartmouthatlas.org/tools/faq) and "Reflections on Variations" (at the link dartmouthatlas.org/keyissues/issue.aspx?con=1338), the Dartmouth researchers cite evidence that regional variation in the rates of common surgical procedures is not explained by differences in socioeconomic or health factors inherent to the populations in those regions. They further state that on average, regions with higher rates of procedures do not show better patient outcomes than regions with lower rates of procedures. They estimate that at least 30% of all clinical care spending could be avoided without worsening health outcomes. (See also the Dartmouth Atlas webpages on "Supply-Sensitive Care", describing how over-supply of medical resources leads to over-utilization.)

Similarly, a 2012 report by the Institute of Medicine (IOM) estimates that a third ($750 billion) of annual US healthcare expenditure is waste, with $210 billion of that waste due to unnecessary medical services (i.e., over-treatment) and $55 billion due to prevention failures.

The recent article, "When Evidence Says No, but Doctors Say Yes", *ProPublica*, Feb. 22, 2017, speaks further to the ubiquity of over-treatment.

Some of the drivers of over-treatment

A major contributor to over-treatment is the prevailing *fee-for-service* payment model (also called *pay-per-procedure*) that we have in the US. In this model, doctors and hospitals charge a fee for each service rendered – office visit, test, procedure – rather than charge a set price for a bundled treatment package. Unfortunately, this paradigm incentivizes doctors to keep office visits short, and order as many tests and procedures as possible. It encourages doctors to deliver volume of care rather than quality of care.

Over-treatment often results from efforts to identify and treat disease in its earliest stages, before evidence has emerged that the disease is progressing and could become dangerous. For example, since July 2012, the US Preventive Services Task Force has been recommending against routine PSA screening for prostate cancer because most tumors found early turn out to be benign, and aggressive treatment often harms patients.

To guard against malpractice lawsuits and liability, many doctors order unnecessary medical tests and over-prescribe drugs. In a 2005 survey, 93% of 824 doctors admitted that they practice "defensive medicine", prescribing unwarranted imaging, biopsies, and medications. Not only is this expensive for the healthcare system, but it can actually pose risks to the patient. (See "Defensive Medicine Among High-Risk Specialist

Physicians in a Volatile Malpractice Environment", *JAMA*, June 1, 2005.)

Patients themselves can drive over-treatment by pressing their doctors for medications and tests that are not warranted. Since insured patients are usually shielded from large out-of-pocket costs, they are incentivized to try any medical service that they think might do some good.

Hospitals – putting the patient at risk

Going into the hospital? Good luck! – you'll need it. That's according to the article, "Medical error – the third leading cause of death in the US", *BMJ*, May 3, 2016. (See also, "Medical Errors Are No. 3 Cause Of U.S Deaths, Researchers Say", *NPR*, May 3, 2016.) More than 250,000 people a year die from medical mistakes at the hospital. What is the nature of these mistakes? They include: failure of coordination in care; poor judgement; insufficient skill; diagnostic errors; wrong drug; wrong dose; bad drug combination; and others. Turns out, the rate of medical errors varies greatly from hospital to hospital, as can be seen from national studies published online by The Leapfrog Group.

Variation in the pricing of medical services

In 2013, the Centers for Medicare and Medicaid Services released data comparing the prices charged for the 100 most common treatments at over 3,000 hospitals across the US. The differences in billing, even among hospitals located in the same city, were astonishing. For some treatments, the discrepancy was more than three-fold, without any evidence that the more expensive hospitals were generating better patient outcomes than the less expensive hospitals. (See, for example, "Hospital Billing Varies Wildly, Government Data Shows", *The New York Times*, May 8, 2013.)

In 2013, CalPERS, the California health plan for state and municipal employees, found a five-fold difference in hospital billing across the state for hip and knee replacement surgery – again, with no evidence of a difference in outcomes. (See the June 18, 2013 notice with item name "Hips and Knees Reference Based Pricing Evaluation" put out by the CalPERS Pension & Health Benefits Committee.)

The FDA – not the guardian you think

The Food and Drug Administration (FDA) is responsible for regulating drugs and devices sold in the US market. It sets the standards for market entry, and does some amount of post-market safety monitoring. In order for a new drug to be sold in the US, it first has to undergo FDA clinical trials that demonstrate safety and efficacy. These trials comprise three phases, ranging in total duration from 2 to 10 years, with an average total duration of 5 years. The FDA has a different approval process for devices. The agency regulates drug manufacturing, distribution, labeling, and advertising. It has the authority to recall drugs and devices when evidence emerges that they are unsafe.

You might think that the FDA is a potent regulatory agency ensuring safe, effective, and even cost-effective medicine. In actuality, the FDA falls well short of that mark. See, for example, "Gaps, Tensions, and Conflicts in the FDA Approval Process: Implications for Clinical Practice", *J Am Board Fam Pract*, Mar-Apr 2004. Today, the situation is no better than it was in 2004, and in some ways it's worse. In general: the FDA sets a low approval bar for drug efficacy; does not compare drugs; does not assess or advise on cost for value; is under-resourced for its tasking (which includes post-market surveillance of more than 5000 drugs, and monitoring of advertising and marketing campaigns); suffers from conflicts of interest; is buffeted by political winds; does not regulate off-label drug prescription; and does not adequately regulate diagnostic "laboratory developed tests". The FDA rarely subjects new devices to clinical trials nor does it regulate new surgical procedures. Often it is too slow to issue recalls of drugs and devices when safety issues arise. It does not provide adequate regulation on herbals and dietary supplements.

So where does this leave us?

In US healthcare, there's a lot of over-treatment, a lot of inappropriate, ineffective, and harmful treatment, and a lot of unnecessary medical tests. This is a reflection of flawed medical decisions, which serve neither patients nor the healthcare system. Clearly what's needed is a rigorous, objective, unassailable methodology for making good medical decisions, decisions most likely to meet the patient's goals. Fortunately, such a methodology exists. It seeks objective understanding of past patient experience and uses it to predict future patient experience. We call the approach *rigorous statistics*. It enables mathematically-supported comparisons among treatment options, allowing for the highest degree of rational choice among those options. We can't tell you what rigorous statistics is right now, but we will do so later, and in enough detail to leave no doubt of the methodology's validity and usefulness.

Ch. 3 Static Thinking in Dynamic Times

To-morrow, and to-morrow, and to-morrow creeps in this petty pace from day to day, says Shakespeare's Macbeth. But in these times, at least in science and technology, we are rushing into the future at such a pace that innovations of one day are eclipsed by those of the next. The explosion in technology has been a boon to engineering, science, electronics, finance, art, entertainment, and medicine. Our smart phones, smart cars, and smart houses keep getting smarter.

On the other hand, some important aspects of medical practice have been slow to change. Although physicians readily embrace devices like the CAT, MRI, and PET imaging machines, and the da Vinci surgical robot, and are quite willing to prescribe new medications on the notoriously untrustworthy advice of drug reps, they have been slow to appreciate the enormous benefits to medical decision-making that would result from widespread, real-time *rigorous statistical analysis* on standardized electronic medical records. (Again, we'll explain what rigorous statistics means later.) Medicine has been slow to enter the Information Age compared to other fields. As a result, today's medical practice is far short of where it should be in terms of delivering best-practice care on a per-patient basis.

Only since 2009, with the American Recovery and Reinvestment Act, did a serious push begin for widespread adoption of electronic medical records (EMR's). This legislation requires that healthcare providers utilize EMR's in a significant way by 2014 or lose their Medicare reimbursements at an increasing annual rate (1% in 2015, 2% in 2016, 3% in 2017) until compliance. Today, compliance exists to a high degree. The initial goals of the legislation were to reduce administrative costs, facilitate sharing of patient information across providers, and promote accurate and up-to-date record keeping. The longer term goal is to use large repositories of EMR's for analysis purposes, use them to identify best-practice medical care. The EMR is ultimately envisioned as a standardized digital record containing the patient's entire medical history across practices. This includes patient demographics, vital signs, current and past symptoms and diagnoses, test results, treatments, doctor's notes, doctors who treated, and hospitals that treated. Getting all these items sufficiently structured and standardized so that the various commercial EMR systems can insert and extract information has been a challenge. But eventually this will happen.

So, why do doctors embrace new surgical and imaging machines so readily, but not the concept of rigorous statistical medical advice or decisions delivered by computer?

One reason is that surgical robots and imaging devices are seen as tools that enhance the physicians existing abilities, extending the physician's reach and senses. They do not challenge the physician's skill, judgment, expertise, or intuition. And they do not shake the patient's view of the doctor as the ultimate medical authority.

Another reason is that physicians are generally not proficient in statistics, a subject not extensively covered in the med-school curriculum. Many physicians do not understand what rigorous statistics is, nor why it is the best way to arrive at patient-centric, medical decisions, better than decisions based on experience, intuition, and supposed knowledge of the patient.

Many physicians fear that computers offering rigorous advice on best-practice medical care will diminish their professional prestige, reduce the number of procedures they perform, subtract from the bottom line, and possibly put them out of a job.

Of course, medicine is not the only bastion of resistance to the idea that machines might be "smarter" than we are in certain domains. Antiquated mindsets are found in all realms. Here are some examples of static thinking.

Conversation with a mathematician and computer scientist

Even before Isaac Asimov's, *I, Robot*, in the 1940's, philosophers and scientists debated the possibility of computer intelligence:

Alan Turing (1912 – 1954), inventor of the *Turing machine* (a mathematical definition of "algorithm"), is considered the father of modern computer science. He not only believed in machine intelligence, but offered the following thought experiment as a vehicle for recognizing it: Imagine a person sitting in a room across the hall from another room. A go-between delivers questions from the first room to the second, and comes back with the answers. Based on these answers, the person in the first room has to decide whether there is an intelligent entity in the second room. Over the years, this thought experiment has produced a mountain of academic papers, and a grand debate as to what constitutes intelligence continues to this day. For the authors of this book, intelligence is as intelligence does. Our definition is operational: If a task is thought to require intelligence, and an entity completes that task, then we see the entity as intelligent – be it man or machine.

Back in the days of Pac Man, in the early 1980's, computer chess-playing programs were introduced that could pose a reasonable challenge to humans. Still, many were not impressed. First they said a computer will never beat a talented eight-year-old. When it did, they said a computer will never beat a talented twelve-year-old. When that happened, they said that no computer will ever beat a national master. Eventually that happened too, and so on.

Of all recreational board games, chess has long been seen as a supreme test of strategic and analytical thinking – a game that requires intelligence, deductive reasoning, and the ability to weigh different options. In 1989, IBM decided to take up the challenge of creating the ultimate chess-playing automaton, and in 1997 reached the goal in spectacular fashion. Their supercomputer, Deep Blue, beat the reigning world champion, Gary Kasparov, and became the new Grandmaster. Shortly afterwards, it was de-commissioned.

People today still play chess against people, but freely-available software running on a PC is able to beat most players at the Master's level, while top proprietary software can defeat World Champion level players.

When Deep Blue became World Champion, a colleague of ours, a professor of mathematics and computer science, asked in casual conversation if the computer exploited some novel kind of algorithm or strategy in its play, a strategy different from that of humans.

The answer was no. Deep Blue basically drew its strength from brute-force computing power and prodigious memory. To initialize the parameters of its play, it started off by analyzing 700,000 grandmaster games. Then during play, it pursued exhaustive search in a game tree that was 10 moves deep, analyzing 200 million board positions per second using massively parallel hardware.

Our colleague was deeply disappointed. To him, Deep Blue did not represent real machine intelligence. Yes, the machine could beat the pants off any human opponent, but that was only because it had access to virtually unlimited speed and memory. "We humans are the intelligent ones," he said, "because even with our limitations, we still manage to put up a good game!"

It's a common human foible: the attitude that if the other solves a problem using resources beyond what we can muster, then the other is "cheating", and should not be considered as intelligent as we are.

Conversation with another mathematician and computer scientist

This conversation took place some fifteen to twenty years ago at a dinner party: The professor was quite certain that pursuing automated language translation was fool's folly. As proof, he told of a program designed to translate from English to Russian and from Russian to English. Given the challenge, "The spirit is willing, but the flesh is weak," the Russian translation came back, "The vodka is strong, but the meat is rancid." Though Dostoyevsky may have said it differently, modern translation programs are infinitely more useful than what we humans can do in real-time with a paper dictionary. Today, translation apps on smartphones are used routinely around the world, and they're getting better all the time.

This highlights another common human foible: the attitude that if the other doesn't perform as well as the very best of us, then it's inferior to all of us.

The professor continued: "Can you tell the difference between a cat and a dog? Well, *you* can but the computer can't." After a pause, we decided not only that the computer could, but could do so even better than the human: If you were to look at someone standing across the room holding a Pekinese in one arm and a Peke-Faced Persian in the other, you would find it very difficult to distinguish the dog from the cat. Some years ago, expert taxonomists had trouble deciding the status of the cheetah – is it a cat, a dog, or something else? The problem is that although the cheetah resembles a cat in most respects, it lacks retractable claws, which at the time, was considered a defining characteristic of cats. Today, after comparing the genomes of cheetahs, cats and dogs, the consensus is that the cheetah is a cat. This example illustrates that computers, using approaches very different from humans, can sometimes resolve questions in a more satisfactory way than humans.

Conversation with a veterinarian

The veterinarian recalled that a decade earlier, one of his professors was working on a computer program to automate semen analysis in order to quantify sperm motility, an important factor in assessing animal and human fertility. After a great deal of effort, the professor saw little progress, and eventually dismissed the idea that sperm motility evaluation would ever be done by machine.

Yet today, automated semen analysis is the norm for assessing fertility – it's almost never left for a human to do. A video processing algorithm can track the motion of each sperm cell over time and determine whether its motion is directed (and purposeful) or undirected.

Conversation with Joe and Jane patient

Ask Joe and Jane on the street what they think of the idea of machines dispensing medical advice in order to guide treatment selection, and you find that many are not so keen on the idea. They don't want to be seen as inanimate data points number-crunched by a cold, emotionless computer. Instead, when they go to the doctor's office, they want to be seen as living, breathing, flesh-and-blood human beings, unique individuals deserving of personalized expert attention. This they believe can only be dispensed by a compassionate, empathetic physician who "understands" them. They argue that a computer can't possibly know the patient.. What Joe and Jane don't realize is that *rigorous statistics* based on computerized analysis of historical patient data can actually deliver *more* personalized and *more* defensible advice than they would get from any doctor.

Conversation with a head-and-neck surgeon

"If something goes wrong in the operating room, it's usually a problem with anesthesia." said the surgeon, and continued. "Anesthesiology is a demanding and stressful specialty. There are so many things to monitor, and so many things that can go wrong, and when something does go wrong, it's often a life or death situation. Every patient is different and you always have to expect the unexpected. Only a human can manage such complexity. No machine could ever do the job."

But wait, isn't this the perfect task for a computer? A computer doesn't tire, can't be distracted, is available 24/7, can react in a blink, and can be programmed to respond to all sorts of rare events. That was our take.

"Preposterous!" said the surgeon.

That conversation took place in 2011. The next day, after Googling "automated anesthesia", we discovered that such a machine, named *McSleepy*, had already been prototyped in 2008 at McGill University, and continues to be tested in real operations. The machine is a fully autonomous anesthesiology robot (except for intubation) that monitors the patient's vital signs in real-time and adjusts the chemical drips accordingly.

Other kinds of automation are heading for the operating room a well. Robots are being developed to operate on the middle and inner ear. The first such machines will work in cyborgian partnership with a human surgeon, but later we can expect the cyborg to evolve more and more into a fully autonomous robot.

Eye surgery, another specialty demanding extreme steadiness and precision, is also looking to machines for help. Some robots are already in use, while others are under active development. Again, the cyborgs will come first, to be followed by more and more autonomous machines.

A practicing surgeon may think that there isn't enough time to learn to partner with a machine. However, it only takes a couple of weeks, for instance, to train a surgeon on a da Vinci robot. This is done using a dual control da Vinci: one set of controls for the student, the other for the teacher, who can override the student's controls if necessary, just like a dual control car for driver training.

The common trend in technology is to shift responsibility from human to cyborg, and then from cyborg to fully autonomous robot or system. In the end, let machines do what machines do best, and let humans do what humans do best. It's a division of labor that will change in time as technology advances.

Most surgeons will adapt and learn to work with machines. Others will stick with the old ways for a few more years until they can slip into a comfortable retirement.

Conversation with an internist

This doctor may be more of a reactionary than most. Forever at odds with the computer, he was particularly annoyed when the hospital where he worked demanded that all physicians train and use a voice recognition system to enter doctor's notes into patients' electronic medical records. "A huge waste of time," he said. "All pain and no gain." And he was certainly dismissive of the possibility that machines could ever play a major role in guiding diagnosis and treatment. He offered the following patient case as an example of human decision-making that he believed was beyond the capability of the computer:

A patient came into his office complaining of severe chest and joint pain. The usual exam showed nothing, and nothing in the patient's medical record offered a clue. The doctor came around to asking the patient what had been going on in his life recently. The patient answered that he had just returned from a scuba diving trip. Bingo! The doctor guessed that the patient might be suffering from the bends (decompression sickness), and sent him over to a facility with a hyperbaric chamber. Turns out, that was exactly what the patient needed. Patient cured! Case closed!

Yes, this was a good call by the doctor, and he is justifiably proud of it. But his claim that a machine could never possess the kind of smarts needed to make such a diagnosis is flat-out wrong. Imagine a computer with access to a database of historical patient EMR's. Suppose the database contains examples of patients who were recorded to have the same symptoms as the bends, as well as a description of events that preceded the symptoms, and evidence that the symptoms were correctly diagnosed as the bends. The machine now has an awareness of the kind of patient just seen by our doctor friend. The computer, by employing a decision tree – akin to one for trouble-shooting a car problem – can determine if the current patient is similar to patients in the database who were correctly diagnosed with the bends. In working through the decision tree, the computer might direct the doctor to collect more information from the patient before offering its diagnosis.

Conversation with a pediatric surgeon

In the middle of the night, many years ago, we found ourselves in the emergency ward speaking with a pediatric surgeon. Our three-year-old son had awakened screaming in pain, his stomach distended and drum-tight. A quick exam led to the diagnosis of intussusception, a fairly rare condition in a three-year-old, where one section of the small intestine engulfs an adjoining section. Blood supply to the engulfed segment is restricted and the latter soon begins to die.

The surgeon said that we had to decide, and decide quickly. There were two choices: operate, or try to relieve the condition by administering a barium enema under pressure. The first meant operating in the intestinal cavity without ideal preparation of the patient for this kind of surgery, entailing a high risk of infection. The second carried the risk of rupturing the intestine, again leaving the patient open to infection. "What do you want to do?" the surgeon asked. "You have to decide now."

Decide now! Well, give us some odds – what is the likelihood of infection for each procedure? What is the probability of success in the short term? The long term? But it was the middle of the night. There was no opportunity for consultations. The numbers we so desperately needed were not available, and we had never heard of the condition before. So we took a guess and decided to go with the barium enema. We were lucky – it worked.

But had the medical community gathered statistics on cases like this, the surgeon would have been in position to advise. Though this episode occurred more than forty years ago, it still represents the kind of situation that can occur today – insufficient access to statistical data when it's urgently needed. In these times, there is no excuse for that.

Visit to the dermatologist

Melanoma is a killer. Early diagnosis is the key to survival. But not every skin spot is melanoma – in fact, few are. So before a biopsy is ordered, the dermatologist will examine the blemish by eye and assess its "ABCDE": **A**symmetry, **B**orders (irregularity of shape), **C**olor (variegation), **D**iameter, and **E**volution (of size, shape, and color over time). If any of these raise suspicion, a biopsy is taken and sent to the lab. A histopathologist examines the biopsy under a microscope and looks for an abnormal distribution of the melanocytes (the melanin-producing cells of the skin). If the distribution doesn't look right, the verdict is melanoma, and the patient is in for some surgery.

And all of this is done by eye and experience. But what's an irregular border? What's a pronounced variegation of color? What's an abnormal distribution of melanocytes? These terms are subjective and imprecise when judged by a human, and sometimes it can be difficult to get two doctors to give the same opinion. It's an archaic way of doing things.

On the other hand, utilizing digital photos of a skin mole, a computer equipped with image processing algorithms can quantify its "ABCDE" in a precise and objective manner. Such software will soon be more reliable than any human dermatologist screening for melanoma. (We'll revisit this topic in Chapter 10.) Eventually, image processing software will do the biopsy analysis itself, and do so more reliably than any human histopathologist.

Everyone has some skin in this game. In the future, whom will you trust to make the best decisions: dermatologists and histopathologists, or the machine?

May the better diagnostician win!

Conversation with a plastic surgeon

"In my profession," the plastic surgeon said, "there is no need for mathematics or statistics."

If a young person has an overshot or undershot jaw, surgical intervention might be called for. The surgeon might remove bone from the mandible in the first case, or slice the mandible and insert a spacer to become bone in the second case. Neither procedure is fun – the patient will certainly not want to revisit the problem again. But bones grow at different rates at different times in a person's life: faster in children, slower in adults; faster in those destined to be tall, slower in short folks.

So there's a problem: How much bone do you remove or add? Many factors have to be considered in order to best suit the needs of the individual. A shattered leg bone or arm bone presents the same sort of problem.

Of course, the surgeon could make the decision just using intuition, experience, and training. But wouldn't it be better to let a computer plan the surgery, using a mathematical formula for bone growth?

The way doctors (shouldn't) think

In his 2007 bestselling book, *How Doctors Think*, Dr. Jerome Groopman inadvertently shows us the way doctors shouldn't think. Dr. Groopman is Chair of Medicine at Harvard Medical School and is Chief of Experimental Medicine at Beth Israel Deaconess Medical Center. He is the author of five books, all written for a general audience, and has published many scientific articles. Of course, he does not speak for all physicians, but his views are widely known and influential, and have remained consistent for the past ten years (as can be seen in recent interviews online). So when he shows a profound lack of understanding of the statistical approach to medical decision-making that medicine so desperately needs in order to advance in the twenty-first century, we have to be concerned. His book describes various case studies of wrong-thinking by doctors, and his cure for their wrong-thinking is more of the same-old-same-old: vague, unfocused, unscientific strategies, bordering on the mystical, with talk of "intuition" and "heuristics", self-reflection, and having special rapport with the patient. Statistical thinking is essentially dismissed as being irrelevant or even counter-productive. His book is part of the problem, not the solution.

The book opens with the case history of a young woman who, beginning in 1990, suffers for fifteen years from a growing list of gastrointestinal problems: initially it was stomach pain and nausea, then intestinal cramps, vomiting, diarrhea, and weight-loss, and eventually severe symptoms of nutritional malabsorption. At first, she was prescribed antacids, which didn't help. Later she lost her appetite, forced herself to eat, then felt sick and purged. She was referred to a psychiatrist, who diagnosed her with anorexia/bulimia and put her on a standard treatment. Her condition worsened. Over the next decade and a half, she ended up seeing thirty doctors (internists, endocrinologists, orthopedists, hematologists, infectious disease doctors, psychologists, and psychiatrists), and was ultimately diagnosed as having irritable bowel syndrome, in addition to the earlier psychological diagnosis. Eventually, down to eighty pounds, she resigned herself to the hopelessness of her condition.

Nevertheless, her boyfriend managed to convince her to seek the opinion of yet one more doctor. This doctor ended up doing something different from all the others. He took her medical record, and instead of scrutinizing it, pushed it to the side, pulled out a notepad and pen, and began interviewing her from scratch and at length. Following that, he then examined her for specific symptoms, ordered blood tests and an endoscopy, and quickly arrived at a totally new diagnosis: celiac disease. And with that, the patient was on the road to recovery.

This doctor, a well-known gastroenterologist, certainly deserves credit for properly diagnosing the patient. So, what were the special abilities that enabled this doctor to succeed where so many others had failed? Dr. Groopman rhapsodizes on them: his ability to recognize and learn from past mistakes; his ability to establish good rapport with the patient; his excellent clinical "intuition" and superb mastery of medical "heuristics"; and his ability to think outside the box.

Of course, there's another moral that could be taken from the story: What was going on in the minds of the previous twenty-nine doctors? How could so many doctors be so ill-equipped to discover what was wrong with the patient?

Perhaps doctors can be trained to have better rapport with their patients and learn to listen better. If doctors have been in practice for a while, hopefully they do build up useful experience and knowledge beyond their textbook training, and hopefully learn from past mistakes. But what about newly-minted doctors who don't have much experience?

What are the definitions of "good clinical intuition" and "correct medical heuristics"? How do you train a doctor to have these skills? How do you confirm that they've been assimilated? Are these skills latent in every doctor, just waiting to be tapped? If so, how long does it take to develop them, and does every doctor need the same amount of time? Should the slow pokes be allowed to practice before the skills are in full bloom, practice at the patient's peril? And if there are those who just can't harness the magic, how do you recognize them, and should they be allowed to practice at all?

And regarding the long-suffering patient who was finally diagnosed correctly as having celiac disease, could not a decision-tree built from a large number of historical patient EMR's (that includes patients who had celiac disease) have directed any doctor to check for specific symptoms, order blood tests and an endoscopy, and homed in on the correct diagnosis from the start? You bet it could!

The following statements (in italics) taken from Dr. Groopman's book express his views on clinical practice:

Clinical algorithms can be useful for run-of-the-mill diagnosis and treatment – but they quickly fall apart when symptoms are vague, or multiple and confusing, or when test results are inexact. (p. 5)

That's totally backwards! It's precisely when the situation is complex, when the symptoms are many or vague, that the computer – armed with standardized EMR's and rigorous mathematical-statistical algorithms – is really going to shine. The simplest cases, requiring only a Band-Aid and chicken soup, can be handled by your mom.

But today's rigid reliance on evidence-based medicine risks having the doctor choose care passively, solely by the numbers. Statistics cannot substitute for the human being before you; statistics embodies averages, not individuals. Numbers can only complement a physician's personal experience with a drug or a procedure, as well as his knowledge of whether a 'best' therapy from a clinical trial fits a patient's particular needs and values. (p. 6)

A computer can search a huge database of standardized EMR's for all historical patients who had the same health complaint as the current patient and were similar in terms of age, gender, race, build, vitals, health history, family history, and so on, even down to the level of values and priorities. From these records, the computer can tell you the statistical performance of each treatment, thereby giving insight into which treatments are likely to perform best for the current patient. The most prodigious human memory and the most extensive human experience are no match for a machine that can access and analyze potentially millions of medical records. Even if the search turned up only a small number of records, the computer, with the tools of statistics, can tell you what conclusions can be drawn from the data and with what confidence.

But few of us realize how strongly a physician's mood and temperament influence his medical judgment. (p. 8)

The great thing about the computer is that it's rarely moody or temperamental, doesn't have off-days and on-days, never gets sleepy, is never influenced by feelings toward the patient, doesn't have a golf game to get to at 5:00 pm, and isn't concerned about the bottom line.

...Bayesian analysis, [is] a method of decision making favored by those who construct algorithms and strictly adhere to evidence-based practice. But in fact, few if any physicians work with this mathematical paradigm. (p. 11)

To the extent that's true, it's detrimental to the practice of medicine. Don't we want our medical care to be as evidence-based as possible, drawing on past patient experience to the fullest degree and employing analyses that are based on rock-solid, mathematics whenever possible?

...[the doctor] should also be schooled in heuristics ... the foundation of all mature medical thinking. (p. 36)

Dr. Groopman never actually defines what "heuristics" is, so it's unclear what is being taught to med students and how they could be tested on it. Wouldn't it be better to teach the aspiring doctor a more rigorous, well-defined, mathematical approach that leverages past patient experience as the primary guide to diagnosis and treatment for the current patient? Using heuristics as a cover for the absence of rigorous exploration and reasoning is shameful.

Dr. Groopman suggests that rigorous statistical analysis on historical patients similar to the current patient can misdirect the doctor's decision-making. This goes completely counter to the idea of evidence-based medicine.

But if the doctor doesn't understand the fundamental concepts of rigorous statistics or can't appreciate its place in medical decision-making, then one of two things will happen: The doctor won't use it, or the doctor will use it but potentially incorrectly, both leading to inferior care for the patient. Not a good model for modern medicine.

We believe that the great majority of doctors and patients are capable of learning the basics of statistics. They don't have to be experts, but a near-total lack of knowledge in this realm is preventing medical practice from moving forward, preventing patients from getting the best care possible. It impedes the drive for better, more cost-effective healthcare.

Battling the old guard

It is difficult to get a man to understand something when his salary depends on his not understanding it.

Upton Sinclair

Sinclair has it right. And it's just as true of image, prestige, and self-esteem. It's not always easy to accommodate change, especially when your livelihood and reputation are grounded in the old ways. And when your profession requires years of study and expense, and the change threatens to make certain aspects of your practice obsolete, many will resist change as forcefully as they can. The concept of and push for evidence-based medicine, medicine based on solid statistical analysis, challenges those in the medical profession to think differently and adjust practice accordingly. Doctors – accustomed to learning more by rote than by reason – more by example than by deduction – may find the statistical approach challenging at first, not having had the training and experience needed to develop this mode of thinking.

Soon, we'll introduce the reader to the basic ideas of *rigorous statistics* in a succinct, understandable, compelling, and useful way.

Ch. 4 Winners and Losers

Patients usually defer medical decisions to their doctors. Doctors generally select treatment based on med-school training, limited personal experience, intuition, heuristics, hearsay, and habit. That decision may be further influenced by stress, fatigue, feelings toward the patient, and concerns about the bottom line. Subjective thinking is a clear danger. That's the way medical decisions are made currently; the way they've been made forever.

But today we can forget this antiquated approach to medical decision-making, and instead, leverage rigorous statistics on standardized EMR's of past patients similar to the current patient. This allows for objective assessment of historical treatment performance, which can be used to identify those treatments that are the most likely to be of greatest benefit. Now that's revolutionary – removing all subjectivity from medical decision-making, except for the patient expressing his personal values and priorities.

Every revolution has its winners and its losers. The revolution we are backing in medical decision-making is no exception. There will be winners and losers – among patients, among doctors, drug manufacturers, device makers, lawyers, insurance companies, hospitals, politicians, and policymakers. Patients who join the revolution will be winners. And so will everyone else who's pursuing better health care at affordable prices.

Patients among the winners and losers

Some patients believe that nothing can substitute for the hands-on ministrations of a compassionate, empathetic physician – the hard-won expertise and intuition of an old-school practitioner. For these patients, the ability to diagnose, recommend treatment, and offer prognosis are uniquely human skills, skills that a machine will never be able to replace.

And yet this mindset has led to high rates of over-treatment, ineffective and harmful treatment, and unnecessary medical tests, as well as high medical costs. Patients who insist on staying with the traditional paradigm will be losers in the quality and cost of their health care.

Other patients will embrace the enormous advantage that computers and data can bring to medical decision-making. They see the machine as the best agent to deliver objective, evidence-based medicine. They recognize the computer as being able to access vast amounts of historical patient data, rigorously analyze that data, and arrive at treatment advice with a level of rigor well beyond that which can be claimed by any doctor. These patients will be winners.

Doctors among the winners and losers

Physicians, with their extensive training, investment of time and money, career prestige, and high compensation, tend to be protective of their turf. On the other hand, they have had little if any training in statistics. Many physicians do not understand what *rigorous statistics* is nor why it is the best way to arrive at patient-centric, medical decisions, better than decisions based on med-school training, limited personal experience, intuition, and presumed knowledge of the patient.

The doctors who see the shortcomings of the traditional paradigm, and are committed to providing the highest-quality, affordable health care to their patients, will be winners because patients will prefer to seek their services over those of doctors whose practices are not up to snuff with the capabilities of the Information Age. Word will get out, and the latter doctors will be losers.

Among the medical specialties that are particularly ripe for automation: anesthesiology, radiology, histopathology, cytopathology, and various kinds of surgery. (There's already an eye surgery called photorefractive keratectomy that's performed by robot.)

For example, computerized image processing algorithms will eventually supplant the human histopathologist by improving the predictive accuracy of tissue analysis in two ways: first by quantifying the visual features in a tissue sample in a precise and objective way; and second by applying statistical analysis to a large number of tissue samples from historical patients in order to obtain optimal numerical thresholds that will be used to decide presence of disease. This will make evaluating a new tissue sample much more rigorous and evidence-based than it is now.

In a similar way, image processing algorithms will eventually supplant the human radiologist when it comes to interpreting radiographic and ultrasound images.

The anesthesiologist of tomorrow is also likely to be a machine, an autonomous robot like McSleepy. The machine will monitor the patient's vital signs and adjust the chemical drips accordingly, while always prepared for the "unexpected" – a challenge for the human, but not for the machine – the machine is cool, quick, and alert under all circumstances.

The poor will be winners

The poor of the world in Africa, Asia, India, the Middle East, South America and, yes, even parts of the US, desperately need a health care revolution. Great progress has been made in controlling AIDS and in combating malaria and other diseases. But poverty denies billions of people access to basic health care. In places like Somalia, Nigeria, Angola, and Chad, life expectancy is only about 53 years. In Australia, Canada, Japan, Europe, and the US, it's above 79 years. It's a vicious cycle: poor health of its citizens hinders a country's ability to pull itself out of poverty; while poverty makes it difficult to provide adequate health care. In many of the poorest regions, there are no doctors and no hospitals. If there's an occasional clinic run by a few medical personnel, the workload is unmanageable and working conditions abysmal.

We can't expect doctors to make the enormous sacrifice required to work in the poorest communities and villages (so, many kudos to Doctors Without Borders). Large hospital centers require lots of money, and poorer governments have other priorities. And, as long as there's no social unrest, rulers of poorer nations have little incentive to bring improved health care to the have-nots.

But even in remote, impoverished places, the revolution in medical decision-making can still help. Even in places without direct access to modern hospitals, advanced medical technology, and drugs, and without access to the Internet, the *mindset* of the revolution still has the power to replace myth and superstition with rigorous, evidence-based, medical decisions.

Witch-doctoring and quackery, even under cover of being traditional medicine, should not be allowed to diminish the lives of those living in the boonies. Denying the poor the benefits of rigorous decision-making is not just unnecessary, it's unconscionable. And in today's world, where so many can travel to distant places and mingle with the indigenous population, relying on local superstition and myth to treat disease may pose an existential threat to all of us.

The threats are there: MERS, SARS, West Nile fever, and others, are waiting to erupt. Many think that the 2014-2016 Ebola outbreak in West Africa brought us to the brink. (As of 2016, there is a vaccine for Ebola, but not yet a cure. The vaccine is being stockpiled and only approved for use in the event of an outbreak. See "New Ebola vaccine gives 100 percent protection", *New York Times*, Dec. 22, 2016.) It is known that the disease is easily spread by contact with blood, sweat, or excrement from the patient or the deceased. Yet, in many parts of the world, in places like Sierra Leone and Guinea, tending to the sick in the traditional way requires hands-on nursing. Burying the dead with due respect and ceremony also requires hands-on ministration. But these practices are contraindicated if the disease is to be contained.

Rigorous, evidence-based, medical practice is desperately needed in such places, but it has to be brought in from the outside. That's a real challenge. Convincing indigenous people that they need to abandon their traditional ways of caring for the sick and deceased, and accept the recommendations of health care workers from outside their town, and possibly even outside their country, is not an easy thing.

So how did the people of West Africa finally deal with the Ebola epidemic? They were coerced by the government there, sometimes by force, to submit to testing, to quarantine, and to sanitary hands-off treatment of patients and the dead. With pressure from the outside, they ultimately learned something about the science and history of the disease.

Of course, it would be great if such coercion weren't necessary. It would be great if communities worldwide had access to computers and the Internet. But even if they did, would they have the education and mindset to make proper use of it for medicine?

Abuses by the legal drug lords

Big Pharma has been known to corrupt the FDA's system for deciding if a drug is safe and effective by withholding the results of negative or inconclusive clinical trials. This can lead to drugs being approved that have hidden health hazards, as occurred with

Avandia (for diabetes), Vioxx (for arthritis pain), and Celebrex (for arthritis pain). After these drugs went on the market, many patients suffered serious harms.

In the US, drug makers are allowed to market directly to the public and to doctors. The only other country that allows this is New Zealand. As a result of direct-to-consumer advertising, patients often pressure their doctors into prescribing expensive new medications, which may be no better than, or even inferior to, existing cheaper medications.

In the US, pharmaceutical companies are allowed to engage in financial relationships with doctors in order to promote their drugs. These relationships may include money for research activities, inducements for prescriptions, speaking fees, meals, and travel. A recent ProPublica analysis showed that doctors who received payments from pharmaceutical companies were significantly more likely to prescribe their drugs. (See "Drug-Company Payments Mirror Doctors' Brand-Name Prescribing," *NPR*, Mar.17, 2016.)

In accordance with the 2003 Medicare Modernization Act (MMA), Medicare (with 55 million enrollees as of 2015) is prohibited from negotiating prices with drug companies, and prohibited from creating a drug *formulary* – a list of drugs demonstrated to have the greatest "bang for the buck" – which could be used to inform patients and doctors about treatment options. In addition, Medicare is required to cover the cost of almost any drug approved by the FDA, no matter how expensive or effective. This impacts taxpayers and patients alike. The patient could have a 20% co-pay on a doctor-prescribed drug that costs $100,000 a year and has a low efficacy rate.

By contrast, Medicaid and the Department of Veterans Affairs *are* able to negotiate prices with drug companies – and they pay about half of what Medicare pays. Some estimate that if Medicare were able to negotiate drug prices, it would save the US healthcare system more than $50 billion a year.

So how did MMA come to pass? Perhaps it's no coincidence

that former congressman Billy Tauzin, chief architect and pusher of the MMA bill through Congress, shortly thereafter took a $2 million-a-year job as president of the top pharmaceutical lobby.

Medicare reimbursement policies encourage doctors to prescribe more expensive drugs. Doctors are allowed to buy drugs wholesale from manufacturers and sell them retail to patients. The single biggest source of income for private practice oncologists is the commission they make from cancer drugs. (See "The Cost of Cancer Drugs", *60 Minutes,* Oct. 5, 2014.) Drug companies report to Medicare the average price that they sell a drug to doctor's offices. By law, Medicare then adds 6% to the reimbursement of those offices. The result is that physicians are incentivized to prescribe more expensive drugs over cheaper drugs, as 6% on an expensive drug is certainly more lucrative than 6% on a cheaper one. Here are some other shenanigans: The drug company says to the doctor, "Buy drug X from us for the standard price of $11,000 and we'll send you a rebate for $6,000". The doctor buys the drug, prescribes it to the patient, then charges the patient's insurance company not $5,000, but $11,000. This is accepted industry practice.

US patent law grants 20-year protection on new drugs, which averages to about 10 years of protection after the drug is approved. During this time, competition from generics in the US market is held at bay. But drug companies know how to game the system and make patent life much longer through strategic filing of patent extensions. An original patent might claim a general compound and a single way of delivering it to treat or prevent a certain disease. Successive patent extensions then claim new formulations, new delivery mechanisms, new uses, and so on. This strategy keeps the generics at bay much longer.

Drug prices are 50-100% higher on average in the US than in all other industrialized countries. (See "Why do Americans spend so much on pharmaceuticals?", *PBS NewsHour,* Feb. 07, 2014.) Big Pharma argues that high US prices are needed to cover the costs of R&D and clinical trials. In fact, drug companies spend far more on marketing drugs than on developing them –

sometimes twice as much. (See, "Big pharmaceutical companies are spending far more on marketing than research", *Washington Post*, Feb. 11, 2015.) With big profit margins, the pharmaceutical industry has become a magnet for Wall Street investors.

Although *rigorous statistics* can't control all of the shady machinations of the drug industry, nor the unscrupulous behavior of some doctors, it can provide incontrovertible evidence as to the relative safety, efficacy, and cost-effectiveness of one drug versus another, or versus an alternate therapy. This will enable patients and doctors to make the most informed decisions about treatment, while reining in costs to the healthcare system.

Chalk one up for the opioid cartel

On Oct 15, 2017, the *Washington Post* published a scathing exposé titled, "The Drug Industry's Triumph Over The DEA", by Lenny Bernstein and Pulitzer Prize winner Scott Higham. The focus of the article is the recent opioid epidemic, and it begins by pointing out that as of April 2016, the opioid crisis had already claimed over 200,000 lives, more than three times the number of US military deaths in the Vietnam War.

The article goes on to describe recent legislation that has been crafted to make Big Pharma, drug distributors, chain drugstores, and certain doctors big winners – and the rest of us losers. The article describes the collusion between these parties, their lobbyists, members of Congress, and former DEA (Drug Enforcement Administration) officials who now work for the drug industry, officials originally hired to protect the public from the very cabal they are now shilling for. The new law is tantamount to government support for drug lords – it prevents the government from regulating the distribution channels for the industry's narcotics.

How to fight these drug lords? We have no grand solution except to suggest that an informed public will know who not to vote for in future elections; know not to vote for politicos in bed with the drug lords. Hopefully that will make a difference. Meanwhile, we have to count ourselves among the losers.

Evidence suggests that the demand for opioid pills is often less about escaping physical pain and more about escaping mental pain. Certainly the chemically-driven, psychological crutch is not new. Alcohol, and illicit drugs like coke, crack, heroin, ecstasy, crystal meth, and marijuana, have for decades been serving those suffering from the pain of life itself, serving those who see the dreary dregs of today offering nothing but more of the same tomorrow. But, what's astonishing today is the terrifying rate at which people are turning to opioids as the crutch of choice, getting hooked, over-dosing, and many times, dying.

A major source of mental pain these days is chronic unemployment, which often leads to feelings of despair and worthlessness. Jobs that once gave people a sense of pride and purpose have long been drying up in many communities. Singer-songwriter Bob Seger speaks to the nostalgia for an earlier time:

> *Back in '55,*
> *We were young and proud,*
> *We were makin' Thunderbirds.*
>
> From the song "Makin' Thunderbirds"

People don't make cars anymore. Today, it's machines that make cars, and all sorts of other things. And there is no pride or paycheck in watching a machine build a car.

In "The Link between Opioids and Unemployment", *The Atlantic*, April 18, 2017, a study is cited, one by the National Bureau of Economic Research, which finds that as jobless rate increases, so does the rate of opioid overdoses – as unemployment rises by 1% in a given county, the opioid death rate rises by 3.6% and emergency-room visits rise by 7%.

What can we do as a society to end or at least stem the opioid crisis? By themselves, medical detox and counseling services are usually not enough to kick the addiction long term – the recidivism rate is discouragingly high. What's really needed is to solve the root causes of the problem – unemployment being the major one. That would go a long way in moving us into the winners column.

Off-label drug use

Off-label drug use (OLDU) refers to the prescribing of medications for conditions or in dosages that have not been approved by the FDA. Since the FDA does not regulate how doctors prescribe medications, doctors are free to prescribe OLDU's as they see fit, as long as it can be "reasonably argued" that it's acting in the best interests of the patient. OLDU occurs in every medical specialty, but is most common among patient populations that are less likely to be included in clinical trials (e.g., pediatric, pregnant, or psychiatric patients). OLDUs are often prescribed with little or no clinical evidence. A 2006 study estimated that among a group of commonly-used drugs, 21% of prescriptions were for off-label use. A 2007 study estimated that 79% of children discharged from pediatric hospitals were taking at least one off-label medication. (See the article "Ten Common Questions About Off-label Drug Use", *Mayo Clin Proc*, Oct. 2012.)

Surprisingly, physicians are not required to disclose OLDU to their patients. The medical community justifies this in two ways (quoting from the above source): (1) *disclosure may unduly frighten patients;* (2) *the extensive burden placed on physicians to constantly review and communicate medication risk and benefit information may divert attention away from other more important patient care issues.*

If a patient believes that he or she was harmed by an OLDU, the doctor may be liable if prescribing the drug represents a "deviation" from standard practice.

Though physicians are free to prescribe OLDUs as they

choose, drug manufacturers and marketers are strictly prohibited from promoting drugs for off-label use, though often that doesn't stop them from doing so. In a number of instances, drug companies have illegally encouraged doctors to use drugs in unapproved ways, resulting in major lawsuits and multi-billion dollar settlements, such as those paid out by GlaxoSmithKline and Abbott in 2012, and by Eli Lilly and Pfizer in 2009.

More recently, lawsuits are being brought against INSYS Therapeutics for their opioid drug Subsys, which is FDA-approved only for cancer patients. The drug can lead to addiction and death if not used properly. The suit alleges illegal off-label marketing to doctors outside the specialties of oncology and pain management, including to general practitioners, neurologists, dentists and podiatrists, whose prescriptions were fueling half the sales of Subsys. Fraud charges are being brought against the doctors who have been top prescribers of Subsys for off-label use.

At least, *rigorous statistics* can inform us about the safety and efficacy of OLDU prescriptions.

Unregulated use of laboratory developed tests

Every year in the US, doctor's offices and hospitals order billions of diagnostic tests in which samples of patient blood or tissue are sent off to laboratories for analysis. The receiving lab is often the one that developed, manufactures, and interprets the test, thus leading to the term "laboratory developed test" (LDT). Doctors and patients assume that these tests results are trustworthy. But that trust is not always well-placed.

This is another realm where the FDA exerts little control. The agency does not review laboratory claims of test accuracy, nor does it require that laboratory research on a test be made public. Meanwhile, there are roughly 11,000 labs offering between 60,000 and 100,000 tests on the open market. (See "Why the

FDA Wants More Control over Some Lab Tests", *Scientific American*, Dec. 2016.)

Within the last few years, a number of these tests have proven faulty, which can lead to serious consequences for the patient. A test may fail to detect a life-threatening condition, which means the patient doesn't seek treatment as needed. A test may show a health problem when one doesn't exist, which means the patient may undergo unnecessary, even dangerous treatment. The FDA has identified 20 different types of lab tests that are particularly troubling, including tests for Lyme disease and whooping cough that show a high rate of wrong answers, as well as tests that are purported to determine a woman's risk for ovarian cancer. (See "Why the FDA Wants More Control over Some Lab Tests", *Scientific American*, Dec. 2016.)

In 2014, the FDA proposed guidelines that would require laboratories to submit evidence of safety and efficacy to the agency before tests can be marketed. Today, the guidelines are still under review. (See webpage "Laboratory Developed Tests" on the website fda.gov.)

Regulation of surgery and devices

The FDA does not regulate surgical procedures. Doctors are free to follow their own inclinations when it comes to recommending surgery. If a surgeon deviates from standard practice and causes harm to a patient, that surgeon may be held accountable in a malpractice lawsuit, but it is the patient who must bring the lawsuit – the FDA and Justice Department don't have the authority to do so – and it is the patient who must cover court costs in case of a loss. In other words, the game is rigged against the patient.

Although the FDA does not regulate surgery, it does regulate implantable devices, but the standards for market clearance are usually much lower than for drugs. When a new device is submitted for clearance, the agency first makes a decision as to whether the device is "low risk", "medium risk", or "high risk", a judgement based on intuition and historical precedent. Devices deemed high risk are required to go through the agency's Pre-Market Approval (PMA) process, which requires clinical trials to demonstrate safety and efficacy. Very few implantable devices are deemed high risk. The great bulk of implantable devices are deemed medium risk or below, and these can be cleared through the agency's *Pre-Market Notification 510(k)* process whereby a manufacturer need only argue "substantial equivalence" to a previously cleared *predicate device*. A device cleared by citing a predicate, can itself be cited to clear a third device, which can be cited to clear a fourth device, and so on.

Remarkably, if the first device in the chain is recalled for safety reasons, the FDA does not automatically put more scrutiny on subsequent devices in the chain. Another concern is the agency's subjective and potentially corruptible judgement in assigning the risk level to a new device.

The 510(k) was introduced as part of the Medical Device Amendments Act of 1976. This law gave the FDA the authority to regulate devices in addition to drugs, and set the FDA's thresholds for market clearance. The legislation was introduced in a timeframe when it was becoming apparent that possibly hundreds of thousands of women were being harmed by the Dalkon Shield (the brand name of an intra-uterine device to prevent pregnancy).

In 2002, the Medical Device User Fee and Modernization Act was passed, enabling the FDA to collect fees from device manufacturers to expedite 510(k) and PMA reviews. These fees, along with similar fees collected from drug manufacturers, have become a large part of the FDA's funding, creating the potential for conflict of interests.

Meanwhile, device manufacturers and venture capitalists, constantly lobby Congress to try to loosen approval standards on all types of medical devices.

In numerous instances, the 510(k) process has allowed

dangerous products onto the market, while a more rigorous, evidence-based approval process might have prevented that. Some of these cases have been big news stories. In 1976, the FDA decided that silicone breast implants were medium-risk devices that could be cleared by the 510(k) process. In 1988, with evidence of increasing complication rates, the FDA required that new designs submit to the PMA process. Finally in 1992, with complication rates climbing still higher, the agency pulled silicone breast implants from the market entirely except for use in special circumstances. More recently, big news stories have focused on vaginal mesh, metal-on-metal hip implants, and heart defibrillators, with many lawsuits still working their way through the courts.

Let's look at what happened with vaginal mesh:

(See "Surgery Under Scrutiny: What Went Wrong with Vaginal Mesh", *WBUR*, Nov. 4, 2011. See also "J&J Mesh Approved by FDA Based on Recalled Device", *Bloomberg*, Oct. 27, 2011.)

Vaginal mesh refers to the device (and procedure) wherein surgical mesh is installed trans-vaginally to treat pelvic organ prolapse (POP) and stress urinary incontinence (SUI). Since the mid 1990's, millions of US women have undergone this procedure – roughly 300,000 women in 2010 alone. In 2005, the FDA began gathering outcome data, and over the next few years discovered increasing rates of serious complications. The most common – mesh erosion through the vaginal wall – which can lead to infection, severe pain, urinary issues, and other problems. Removing the mesh is often very difficult and can require multiple surgeries. Since 2009, various studies point to mesh erosion rates as high as 15%. Companies that manufacture and market vaginal mesh are now facing a mountain of lawsuits from women who were injured by their products.

In 1996, the first vaginal mesh product for SUI was cleared through the 510(k) process. In 1999, that product was recalled due to a high rate of complications. In 2002, the first vaginal mesh product for POP was cleared through the 510(k) process, by citing substantial equivalence to, of all things, the 1996 device. Shortly thereafter, other vaginal mesh devices were similarly cleared. Soon entire mesh "kits" were introduced that included tools to aid in the insertion of the mesh. This made mesh installation more straightforward and accessible to general gynecologists, most of whom are not trained in pelvic surgery. Dollar signs were flashing in their eyes. With almost no outcomes data available with which to counsel patients, transvaginal mesh repair took off. Everyone was making money – the device manufacturers, the investors, the doctors. It was so lucrative, that even the most prominent gynecological organizations were reluctant to admit the unsupported nature of the procedure in their clinical practice bulletins.

Then in 2008, the FDA issued its first public health alert, stating that transvaginal mesh repair for POP and SUI can lead to serious complications, though rarely. In 2011, the FDA did an about face, saying that serious complications from transvaginal mesh repair for POP are *not* rare, and that it's unclear whether the procedure is more effective than traditional non-mesh repair, and exposes patients to greater risk. Finally in 2016, the FDA decreed that all new mesh products related to transvaginal repair of POP must submit to the PMA process.

All sorts of surgeries are performed daily: tonsillectomies, C-sections, gall-bladder removal, joint replacements, back surgery, hand and foot surgeries, heart surgeries, mastectomies, and prostatectomies, among the many. There is very little to ensure that these interventions are not being over-recommended by doctors.

Since the FDA doesn't regulate surgery and does such a poor job of regulating devices, it's up to patients to determine whether or not surgery is the best course of action versus other options, and if it is, which surgery. And if a device is involved, which device. *Rigorous statistics* can shed a lot of light on these questions, and promote good decisions.

Boost to your health with dietary supplements?

Dietary supplements, including herbals, are a multi-billion dollar industry separate from the pharmaceutical industry. About 85,000 different dietary supplements are sold in the US today. Major players in the industry have deep pockets and employ their own legions of lobbyists to do their bidding. Consumers should be aware that dietary supplements are not subject to the same degree of scrutiny as prescription and over-the-counter drugs – FDA clearance on efficacy and safety are not required for a supplement to be marketed and sold in the US. The only requirements are good manufacturing practices and accurate content labeling. Even this is difficult to enforce with so many products being offered and only about 25 employees at the division of the FDA that monitors the industry. (For an eye-opening report on dietary supplements, exploring safety, efficacy, regulation, and corporate influence, see the *PBS Frontline* episode "Safety and Supplements", produced in cooperation with the *New York Times*, which aired on Jan. 19, 2016.)

Proponents of herbal supplements argue that herbals are time-honored – that their efficacy and safety have been well-established through a long history of use in folk medicine. They argue that herbals, being natural, are better for you than synthesized chemicals. Natural they may be, but the authors are reluctant to quaff a goblet of hemlock or roll about in a bed of poison ivy.

There are several reasons to be concerned about the efficacy and safety of packaged herbals. Here are a few:

- Lax control over product content is a continuing problem. What's on the label is not always what's in the bottle, and that can be hazardous to your health.

    In early 2015, a massive herbal supplement scam was uncovered involving dishonest labeling of store-brand products sold by GNC, Target, Walgreens, and Wal-Mart.

Many of these products were missing the plant materials on the label, and contained potential allergens that were not on the label.

In late 2015, the US Justice Department filed criminal charges against USPlabs LLC, which at the time manufactured the best-selling workout supplement, Jack3d. It's alleged that the company used a synthetic stimulant made in China to give Jack3d its kick, as well as another of their products, OxyElite Pro, but told retailers that the supplements were made from plant extracts. Dozens of liver injuries were linked to OxyElite Pro with some consumers requiring liver transplants.

The Federal Trade Commission is pursuing other lawsuits against other manufactures for deceptive and potentially dangerous representation of their products.

- The percentage of active ingredients in the herbal does not necessarily agree with the percentages on the label, posing the risk of under-dosing or overdosing.

- Herbals are often hyped without strong objective evidence of efficacy.

- An herbal might be effective and the labeling might be correct, but if the user is taking it in addition to another drug, there is the danger of an overdose or adverse interaction. Even combinations like grapefruit juice plus statin drug or spinach plus blood thinner can be deadly. (For others, Google "drug-herb interactions").

We are not suggesting a ban on dietary supplements, but we are suggesting that consumers have the right to be informed on the potential risks and benefits associated with them. *Rigorous statistics* can really help.

Recreational drug use

If the readers knew our concerns about recreational drugs, the reader might think, "Gee, these guys are no fun at all." But we are not prohibitionists. What others put in their bodies is none of our business – unless we have to pay for it with our tax dollars or health insurance premiums. However, we do feel strongly that people should have adequate information in order to make sensible decisions. Let *rigorous statistics* tell us the personal and societal consequences of consuming booze, caffeine, cigarettes, and e-cigarettes, as well as recreational drugs like weed, cocaine, crack, smack, crystal meth, and whatever else the public is popping, dropping, snorting, or shooting up at the moment. And let's examine these drugs with respect to addiction, long- and short-term health risks, rehab cost, recidivism rate, employability of the user, and overall social consequences. Let's see how nations compare on the effectiveness of prohibition, cost of treatment, and drug availability. Isn't this the kind of information that the medical community, policy makers, and citizens, should know? We need reliable numbers in order to act sensibly.

Ch. 5 The Future Starts Today

Prediction is very difficult, especially about the future.

Niels Bohr

Difficult it may be, but prognostication can also be great fun. In the realm of medicine, just imagine a nanotech *Fantastic Voyage* to the remotest recesses of the human body, lasers blazing away, zapping malevolent microbes at every turn. Or imagine ourselves as ageless creatures, replacing our worn out parts with bright and shiny new parts, healthy and spry forever.

It took considerable restraint, but the authors decided to forego sci-fi visions of what future medicine might look like. There's enough excitement in seeing what computers and automation are capable of today, and reflecting on what that suggests for medicine tomorrow, that it makes fanciful speculation totally unnecessary. So we'll just keep it real, with only an occasional foray into the sphere of pie-in-the-sky.

Thanks to major advances in computer processor speed, chip memory, data storage and retrieval capability, and algorithm design, the power of today's automation is unprecedented

For the last fifty years, computer speed has improved in accord with *Moore's Law* – doubling roughly every two years as the capability to miniaturize and cram more transistors on a chip keeps marching ahead. The trend is expected to continue until around 2025. Today, the processing core for a standard personal computer can execute on the order of 100 billion instructions per second.

At the same time, the ability to store data on ever more compact and cheaper media has also advanced rapidly. In 2000, it was estimated that the text in all 26 million books of the Library of Congress represented about 10 terabytes of uncompressed data. Today, all that data could be placed on about a dozen hard drives with total volume equal to that of a shoebox, and for the price of about $120. Remember when a set of *Encyclopedia Britannica* cost $1,500 (and even more for the gold-leaf, leather-bound edition)?

And now with cloud storage, memory is virtually limitless, and readily accessible even from a smart phone. It will soon be possible to digitally archive the 725 Megabyte genome (that's 2.9 billion base pairs representing 25,000 protein-coding genes) of *every* living person on the planet, along with their health records. So the innermost you can be on file and at your fingertips 24/7 anywhere in the world you may find yourself.

That I should lose to this idiot!

Aron Nimzowitsch, chess master

So shouted Nimzowitsch, as he jumped on the table, about to lose a championship chess match to Frederic Samish in 1923.

Seeing as computers now beat us in a variety of games, and seeing as computers and robots keep taking our jobs, there are those of us who might shout in frustration: *That I should lose to this idiot machine!*

In 1997, IBM's Deep Blue computer beat Gary Kasparov to become world chess champion, even though the damned idiot machine never read a treatise on chess strategy by Aron

Nimzowitsch or Bobby Fisher, or anyone else. Mostly, it just tapped into superhuman speed and memory and applied it in brute-force fashion – nothing resembling new insight or creativity – to beat the pants off all comers of the human sort. Idiot machine!

In 2011, another idiot machine, IBM's Watson, beat the reigning *Jeopardy!* champion. In 2015, Google DeepMind announced software that learns by observation to play a mean game of Space Invaders, comparable to the best humans. In 2016, Google DeepMind's machine learning program, AlphaGo, beat the world champion in the ancient Chinese game of Go, a board game far more complex than chess, with more combinations of moves than there are atoms in the universe. In 2017, Carnegie-Mellon demonstrated a computer program, Libratus, that was able to beat some of the world's top poker players. Other idiot machines work for the big banks, playing a high speed game of stock market.

Computers are getting smarter in other ways. In 2012, Google DeepMind announced a machine that taught itself to recognize cats in YouTube videos. In 2014, Facebook's DeepFace machine learning software showed itself to be as good as humans at recognizing faces in photographs. In 2018, machine learning programs are being used to automatically detect features in satellite imagery, features such as cars, buildings, roads, boats, and so on.

Smartphone apps serve as personal digital assistants, and perform automatic speech recognition, handwriting recognition, and language translation.

Enable a computer to take action and you have a robot. Today, robots do much of our heavy lifting, manufacturing, and assembly. Robots build our cars and build our airplanes. At the same time, cars and airplanes have become much like robots themselves. Smart cars are on the way that will do all the driving while you read the daily news. Commercial jets fly auto-pilot most of the time; and stealth military jets, with their strange angular shapes, are so unstable that flight has to be done by computer. There are robots you can buy that will cut your grass and sweep your floors by themselves, while you sit back and drink an iced tea. New agriculture robots with advanced vision systems can automatically discern weed from crop, delivering a spritz of fertilizer, pesticide, or herbicide on a per-plant basis. Robots ramble around on the surface of mars and in the depths of oceans. They guide the optics and tracking motion of the most powerful telescopes, enabling us to see back to the first moments of time.

Recent advances in autonomous, robot motion-control are astonishing. A 2008 YouTube video from Boston Dynamics shows the four-legged robot, Big Dog, navigating over rough terrain, at one point recovering from a fall on the ice, and at another, recovering from a kick to the side. A 2017 YouTube video from the same company shows the Atlas humanoid robot jumping on boxes and doing backflips.

Yes, the robots are coming. We build them and give them purpose, and then they turn around and take our jobs, working tirelessly 24/7, without pay, and without complaint. But as certain jobs are given over to machines, there will be new opportunities for employment using that technology. So, let's have more of robots – especially in medicine.

Da Vinci surgical robots are already putting in long hours at the operating room. McSleepy, the autonomous anesthesiology robot, is soon to follow, as well as its cyborg sidekick, the Kepler intubation robot. Robotic ear surgeons and eye surgeons are just about ready to go. Computerized monitoring devices already serve duty watching over the recovering patient with complete attention and diligence. Automated endoscopy and colonoscopy will check us out from top to bottom. Even cardiac procedures like ablation will become more and more automated. All of this will be to the benefit of patients.

Micro-technology is being used in the development of brain implants to control epileptic seizures, depression, anxiety, and memory loss, and to restore motor skills. Brain-machine interfaces (BMI) are being developed that allow patients to control robotic limbs with their minds. Maybe someday a microchip inserted in the brain will control hunger, pain, and aggression. This recalls the classic 1950's experiment of Olds and Milner that got mice working their tails off in order to get an electric shock to the limbic region – the "pleasure center" – of the brain. *Brave New World*!

Pacemakers with heart monitors are in wide use, as are insulin pumps that autonomously monitor and deliver insulin for diabetics. Implanted devices can record heartbeat, pulse rate, blood pressure, and blood sugar.

Is there no end to the idiot machine's chutzpa? Could it be that the next thing it will be doing is diagnosis, advising on treatment selection, interpreting radiologic images and histopathology slides, and directing robotic surgery and anesthesia? You bet!

Mapping the inner you

Genes may not be destiny, but often they can warn of potential medical problems, everything from heart disease, diabetes, cancer, to autism, bipolar disease, and many more. A certain genetic profile might predict a disease with absolute certainty, but more often, the prediction is probabilistic. Knowing your genome can give you just the warning you need to try and avoid illness. If, for example, your genetic profile places you at increased risk for heart disease, you might take that as advice to watch your diet and increase your exercise.

With about 25,000 protein-coding genes, it's a good bet that each of us has some bad genes. Some people might prefer not to know of such hidden time-bombs. Others will want to be informed. An unfavorable genetic profile for breast cancer might motivate a woman to get a breast exam with greater frequency, or even undergo a preventive double mastectomy. An unfavorable profile for prostate cancer might convince a man that more radical therapy is more prudent than watchful waiting or active surveillance.

These days, your genome can be commercially sequenced for under $1000 and burned onto a thumb drive. In fact, there are several firms doing just that for their clients now. The service includes flagging individual genes and gene-combinations associated with various diseases – the client can choose not to be informed of such trouble spots, while leaving access to such information to medical professionals.

When it comes to the correct dosage of a medication, one size does not fit all. "Take two pills and call me in the morning" may work for Joe and Jane average, but not so much for the rest of us. Differences in age, sex, weight and many other factors might peg the "standard" dose as an overdose for some and an under-dose for others. In addition to these outwardly-obvious physical factors of a patient, there are a host of invisible genetic factors that may influence the effectiveness of drugs in the treatment of cancer, cardiovascular disease, infectious disease, metabolic disease, depression, bipolar disorder, and many others. Pharmacogenomics is a promising, new, interdisciplinary field combining pharmacology and genetics to individualize drug therapy through knowledge of the patient's genome.

Game On!

Computers and the Internet enable what's called *crowdsourcing*, which can be used to tackle large or difficult problems.

In one version of crowdsourcing, the "leader" partitions a problem into many sub-problems. These are tasked through the Internet to an online community who solve the sub-problems and communicate the solutions back to the leader. The leader then combines these solutions into a solution for the original problem.

Another strategy for crowdsourcing is to invite the online community to solve the same problem (no partitioning) in a sort of competition. Several years ago, gamers everywhere were invited to tackle a problem in protein-folding that had confounded biochemists for a decade. "Online Gamers Crack AIDS Puzzle" –

the headline read. Originally reported in the Sept. 2011 issue of *Nature Structural & Molecular Biology*, it took online gamers only ten days to discover the 3-dimensional folding pattern of an enzyme that is crucial to the development of a virus similar to HIV. The gamers, with no knowledge of biochemistry, played *Foldit*, a program that allowed them to explore the folding patterns of molecules.

The medical implications of such an approach are enormous, not only for HIV, but for any disease that requires an enzyme in order to proliferate – in other words, almost all viral diseases. Disable the enzyme and you block the disease process it catalyzes. But disabling an enzyme usually requires knowing more than its molecular formula. You need to know its geometric structure, its 3-dimensional folding pattern. And that's what the gamers playing *Foldit* discovered – they found the folding pattern of the challenge enzyme. It's a magnificent accomplishment.

The researchers who posed the problem were clever enough to conceive the game *Foldit*, rephrasing a highly technical problem in non-technical terms, presenting it as an understandable challenge to online gamers. We expect this kind of approach to be used more and more to solve problems in the chemical, biological, and medical sciences.

Too exciting not to mention

We don't know to what extent the computer is playing a role in the following research, but here are some recent developments in molecular medicine that are too exciting not to mention in a chapter whose theme is "the future starts today".

Progress is being made towards developing a "universal flu vaccine", a vaccine that can confer protective immunity through multiple flu seasons. Here's the idea: Flu virus looks like a ball with "lollipops" sticking out in all directions. Every year, the proteins that make up the "candy part" of the lollipops change, necessitating a new vaccine to stimulate different antibodies. But the "stem part" of the lollipops does not change – and new stem-targeted vaccines seek to exploit this vulnerability. (See, "A universal flu shot may be nearing reality", *Science News*, Oct. 28, 2017.) We wonder if this approach could be used against other viruses.

Researchers have discovered that a single gene controlling one of the body's "sodium channels" occurs mutated in one way in patients with erythromelalgia ("Man on Fire Syndrome") that are hyper-sensitive to pain, and mutated in a different way in patients with congenital insensitivity to pain. This suggests that a single gene could possibly be manipulated to control pain. (See, "End Pain Forever: How a Single Gene Could Become a Volume Knob for Human Suffering", *Wired*, April 4, 2017.)

Another development focuses on a treatment for Hunter syndrome, a genetic disease that causes developmental delays, organ problems, brain damage, and early death: Recently, gene-editing tools were used *in vivo*, injected directly into a living person. The tools here were designed to target liver cells, splicing in a new gene that can then be chemically controlled to override the defective gene responsible for Hunter syndrome. (See, "A human has been injected with gene-editing tools to cure his disabling disease", *Science*, Nov. 15, 2017.)

Another in vivo genetic therapy, Luxturna, was recently approved by the FDA to treat a certain kind of inherited vision loss that can result in blindness. The treatment involves injecting modified viruses directly into the eye to deliver corrected genes to the retina. Two other *ex vivo* genetic therapies were also approved recently: Yescarta for certain types of lymphoma, and Kymriah for certain types of leukemia. These therapies involve extracting cells from the body, modifying them genetically in the lab, and reinserting them back into the body.

A revolution in medical thinking

Even though some aspects of medicine move forward in lock-step with advancing technology, medical decision-making is stuck in the past, in an outmoded paradigm where doctors still select treatment based on limited personal experience, med-school training, intuition, habit, heuristics, and hearsay, and pressures to feed the bottom-line. It's a mode of decision-making that is subjective and prone to corruption.

Though the medical profession and some patients are reluctant to admit that a computer can deliver better information, better advice, and often better decisions than any doctor, this mindset is at odds with what current technology tells us is possible. In all sorts of applications outside medicine, machines arrive at superior decisions and take superior actions. Clearly, we have the means to deliver patient-centric, evidence-based medicine, by employing rigorous, computerized, statistical analysis of historical patient data. This would be a momentous revolution in medical decision-making.

Ch. 6 Medical Decisions in the Face of Uncertainty

You might think that eons of evolution would have prepared us to cope with uncertainty. But that's not the case, or at least not very well. For many of us, reasoning about risk and chance is difficult, and we are not very good at it. We are easily duped into making bets that are likely to work against us. This is particularly true when faced with decisions about health, when hope and desperation often rule our thoughts. But even with a clear head, probability is a tricky study, full of subtleties that often run counter to our intuitions. And when that happens, some loony part of our brains kicks in to deny the odds, overriding critical reasoning with wishful thinking and notions of being exempt from chance.

Denying that chance rules our lives creates profound misunderstandings about how the world works. Often we imagine that the universe follows laws of our own invention: The roulette wheel stopped on red four times in a row – high time for black. Four sons and no daughters – our next kid will be a girl, for sure. I'm young and healthy and have never been seriously ill or injured, so why should I buy health insurance?

There are many who actually seek out risk, acting in denial, ignorance, or indifference to the odds of a bad thing happening. Some go for the endorphin rush. Others feel that only by taking risks can you truly appreciate life. Some conflate risk-taking with audacity and courage. Let's go BASE jumping. Bungee jumping. Forget the helmet. Forget the ropes. Climb free.

For some, flirting with risk is an uncontrollable urge, as with compulsive gamblers. Then there are those who are too lazy or too lame to weigh the risks. For many though, there is at least some thought given over to risk versus benefit, or risk versus rush. And if the risk to life or limb is minimal, who's to say what's reasonable behavior and what's not? It may just depend on the person's values and priorities. But, if the rest of us have to pay for the reckless behavior of others, or their behavior is a threat to our own health and well-being, that's a different story.

With a general distrust and disregard for all statistics, and a lack of understanding of even the most basic concepts of probability, most people are ill-equipped to make rational decisions in the face of uncertainty. And when it comes to decisions affecting health, being ill-equipped to sensibly judge the options increases the likelihood of a poor outcome. Knowing a bit about probability and statistics can go a long way in decreasing that likelihood. Though they don't grant certainty, probability and statistics are the best defense we have to cope with uncertainty.

By the numbers

Buying a home is a gamble, and most of us look for numbers to help us make the decision: Is the price of the house too dear for this neighborhood? What is the current mortgage interest rate? Is it on the rise or decline? And it's not just buying a home that prompts questions about numbers. They come up when shopping for a car, a major appliance, an education, insurance, investments, and even placing a bet on a sporting event.

Doesn't your health deserve at least as much consideration? Wouldn't you want some numbers, some statistics, before deciding on which treatment to go with? Wouldn't you want answers to questions like: What are the odds this treatment will help me? How much will it help me? How well do we know those odds? What are the odds this treatment will harm me? How much will it harm me? How well do we know those odds? How does this treatment compare to that treatment?

Of course you would, but which statistics? The answer is *rigorous statistics* – unbiased, objective, transparent – based on a foundation of incontrovertible mathematics. We'll explore this framework shortly.

Slow down

I took a speed-reading course and read War and Peace in twenty minutes. It's about Russia.

Woody Allen

If you pride yourself on being a speed-reader, then Part 2 of this book might prove challenging – it's not about Russia. Rather it's about probability, statistics, and getting reliable insights into the world through analysis of empirical observations.

Understanding that "math-speak" is not everybody's idea of poetry, we tried to avoid technical jargon as much as possible. But sometimes special terms and symbols were necessary to avoid excessive verbiage. In line with "keeping it real", we also included many examples of medical significance.

So in going on to Part 2, slow down. Take your time and savor some of the most profound insights by some of the greatest minds of all time – insights that have enabled us to understand the way the world works as deduced from empirical observations and the mathematics of probability.

Part II

In the Face of Uncertainty

Ch. 7 What are the Odds?

To decide what one should do to obtain a good or avoid an evil, it is necessary to consider not only the good and the evil in themselves, but also the probability that they happen or not happen; and to view geometrically the proportion that these things have together.

Port-Royal Logic 14, 16, 1670

Few things in life are certain, and that is certainly true in medicine. From diagnosis to prognosis to predicted outcome of treatment, you often can't know the answers for sure: Do I have condition A or condition B? How will this condition unfold over time? Will the tumor be slow-growing and harmless, or fast-growing and dangerous? Is it better to treat aggressively or take a wait-and-see approach? Is it better to treat with intent to cure or intent to control? Is it better to medicate or operate? Will this treatment harm me? Am I better off taking this drug, that drug, or no drug? Will this joint replacement last me for ten years or not?

But even if the answers are uncertain, you still have to make a decision. You still have to go with something. You take a chance, a gamble. But as with most big decisions, it's a good idea to know the odds before you place your bet, know the probabilities involved. And though the mathematics of probability doesn't grant certainty and doesn't necessarily tell us what we should do, it's the best tool we have to cope with uncertainty – the best tool we have for rational decision-making.

Unfortunately, probability is not the easiest concept to grasp and reason about. Many people find it challenging, unintuitive, and even counterintuitive. But those without at least a minimal understanding of probability (and statistics) are not prepared to be smart consumers of health-related products and services, and are less able to make decisions that best meet their needs and goals.

The probabilistic view can be your friend

Even if a situation is essentially deterministic, it is often more convenient and useful to think of it probabilistically. For example, suppose we flip a fair coin. If we know precisely its initial location and orientation, its exact shape and density, the force used to flip it, the air resistance, and the properties of the surface it will land on, then we can say with absolute certainty whether it will come up heads or tails. However, these particulars are not usually known, nor is it convenient to try and get them. Even if they were known, it would still be a complicated matter to deduce the outcome of the experiment. So, for practical reasons, we model the experiment probabilistically and assume that the coin will land heads one-half the time on average.

Similarly, when tossing a fair die, we adopt a probabilistic model and assume that any face of the die will show itself one-sixth of the time on average.

What about the biological world? Let's recall the work of Father Gregor Mendel, the Austrian monk who created a simple probabilistic model to predict the outcomes of pea-breeding experiments: cross heterozygous *Aa* with homozygous recessive *aa*, and you get 50% *Aa* and 50% *aa*; cross *Aa* with *Aa*, and you get 50% *Aa*, 25% *AA*, and 25% *aa*. On average, that is. When Mendel compared the results of his experiments to those predicted by his model, he reported good agreement. In fact, given today's understanding of probability, we see that his results were a little *too* good – it appears the crafty monk was so confident in his model that he fudged the data to get an even more perfect fit!

Much scientific, medical, and actuarial research involves estimating probabilities. Drug companies have to assess probable efficacy and safety through clinical trials before the FDA will grant approval on a new drug. Genetic counselors have to know the probabilities of genetic diseases before they can provide useful information to their clients. Insurance companies have to know the probabilities of adverse events in order to predict payouts and set premiums. Doctors and patients should understand how to interpret probabilities in order to determine which treatments are most likely to benefit the patient with respect to patient goals.

Benjamin Franklin said it: *In this world, there is nothing certain but death and taxes*. There's truth to that. And though we have to cope with risk and uncertainty every day, mostly we just bumble through it, making decisions that often don't serve us well because we don't grasp the odds. Probability is a subtle topic, often battering our intuitions and leaving common sense in the dust. Nowhere does uncertainty bedevil us more than in health care, where decisions that don't properly recognize risks and probabilities can profoundly impact our health, longevity, quality of life, and wallet. In general, doctors and patients know far too little about probability to deliver and receive the best medical care. We hope to change that here.

Probability by counting

In many practical situations, the appropriate way to compute the probability of something happening – an event – is to use *probability by counting*.

Example 1. Marbles in a hat: Suppose n marbles are in a hat, k of them white and the others black. If you select a marble at random from the hat, then the probability of drawing a white marble is k/n. In other words, you count the number of ways of choosing a white marble and divide by the number of ways of choosing a marble.

Example 2. Tossing a fair die: When tossing a fair die, six outcomes are possible, all equally likely: the face values 1, 2, 3, 4, 5, or 6. So the probability of any specific face coming up is 1/6. In particular, the probability of a 3 coming up is 1/6. Likewise, the probability of a 4 coming up is also 1/6. If you want to know the probability that an even number comes up, a 2, 4, or 6, then that probability is 3/6, which equals ½.

Example 3. Craps: The "shooter" tosses two fair die, say a red one and a blue one. There are 36 possible outcomes, all equally likely, and each outcome can be denoted by a pair (r, b), where r is the face of the red die and b is the face of the blue die. So, the probability of any particular outcome, such as (4, 2), is 1/36. Since there are only two ways of getting a sum of eleven, namely (5, 6) and (6, 5), the probability of tossing an eleven is 2/36, or 1/18. Since there are six ways of getting a sum of seven, the probability of tossing a seven is 6/36, or 1/6. So the event "seven-come-eleven", where either a seven or an eleven is tossed, can occur in 6 + 2 = 8 different ways and so has probability 8/36 = 2/9. Additionally, the probability of tossing "snake eyes" (two ones) is 1/36, and the probability of tossing "box cars" (two sixes) is also 1/36.

Now don't go running off to Vegas just yet – there's a lot more to know about shooting craps. But all of the relevant probabilities are known, easy to compute, and readily available online. Computer programs now play craps as well as any human. Of course, the house always wins in the long run. And of course, if you look online, you will find all sorts of bogus schemes to beat the house. Mark Twain was right in saying: *No one ever went broke betting on the ignorance of the American people.*

A bit of symbology: Sometimes a little symbology can reduce verbiage and enhance clarity:

The set of all possible outcomes of an experiment is called a **population**, which we denote by G. In Example 1, the population G is the set of all marbles in the hat, and the experiment is a random draw from the hat. In Example 2, the population G is the set of all possible face values of the die, namely, $\{1, 2, 3, 4, 5, 6\}$, and the experiment is a toss of the die. In Example 3, the population G is the set of all pairs (r, b), where r is the face value of the red die and b is the face value of the blue die, and the experiment is a toss of both dice.

Any subset of the population G is called an **event**, which we often denote by E, but sometimes other symbols will be used. An event might contain zero, one, or many outcomes, or could even be G itself. In Example 1, the event E of interest is the subset of marbles that are white. In Example 2, one event we considered was the singleton subset $E = \{3\}$. Another was the singleton subset $E = \{4\}$. And another was the subset $E = \{2, 4, 6\}$. In Example 3, one of the events we considered was "sums to eleven", which is the subset of pairs $E = \{(6, 5), (5, 6)\}$. We considered several other events there as well.

The number of members belonging to a finite set X is denoted $n(X)$. The **probability of an event** E is denoted $P(E)$. When using **probability by counting**, we set $P(E)$ equal to $n(E)/n(G)$. This is the appropriate way to compute the probability of an event E when all outcomes in the finite population G are equally likely. In Example 3, all outcomes are equally likely, and so the event "sums to eleven", that is to say, the event $E = \{(6, 5), (5, 6)\}$, has probability $P(E) = 2/36$.

Example 4. Many tosses of a fair coin: Suppose we toss a fair coin ten times. Then the population G consists of all head-tail sequences of length ten. How many such sequences are there? The first toss can land in one of two ways; same for the second; same for the third, and so on. So the number of possible sequences is 2 times itself 10 times, which is 2^{10}, or 1024, and all sequences are equally likely.

If E is the event that no head comes up, then $P(E) = n(E)/n(G) = 1/1024$. That's because only one sequence of length ten is free of heads. If E is the event that exactly one head comes up, then $P(E) = n(E)/n(G) = 10/1024$. That's because there are ten sequences of length ten that have exactly one head.

Suppose E is the event that exactly three heads come up in ten tosses. The number of such sequences in E is 120 (using the proven formula "m choose n" readily available online, and plugging in $m = 10$ and $n = 3$). So the probability of the event E in this case is $P(E) = n(E)/n(G) = 120/1024$.

Example 5. Poker: Perhaps poker is your game. You know when to raise and you know when to fold. You can bluff, and you can call a bluff. Still, it's nice to know a few probabilities.

Let's say you're playing with a standard 52-card deck and you're dealt a poker hand of five cards. Suppose you want to know the probability of being dealt a "royal flush" – that's a ten, jack, queen, king, and ace, all in the same suit. Since there are four suits, the event E of interest contains four royal flushes. How many five-card hands are there? Exactly 2,598,960 (again using the formula "m choose n", but now with $m = 52$ and $n = 5$), Since all 5-card hands are equally likely, the probability of being dealt a royal flush is $P(E) = n(E)/n(G) = 4/2,598,960$, quite a small number.

Want some online tutoring? The computer can help you become a formidable poker player. Not only will it give you the odds of possible hands, but it will provide you with a tireless opponent to play against – one with the perfect poker-face. Don't even try to bluff – it won't work. In 2017, the computer began beating the best poker professionals in the world.

Example 6. Drug dilution schedule: The prescription was for 30 mg capsules of Cymbalta. The doctor had the patient increase the dosage in steps: on days 1, 2, and 3, take a third of a capsule each day; on days 4 and 5, take half a capsule each day; for all days thereafter, take a full capsule. To get the one-third dose, the instructions were to break open the capsule, stir the contents into applesauce, and eat a third of the applesauce each of days 1, 2, and 3. To get the one-half dose, stir the contents of the capsule into applesauce, and eat half the applesauce each of days 4 and 5.

Let's look at this more closely. Each capsule contains six micro-tablets that do not dissolve in applesauce. What is the probability of getting the right dilution on days 4 and 5? The answer is only about 31%! That is to say, only about one-third of the time would you get the recommended three micro-tablets on both days.

Where does this number come from? Imagine that the micro-tablets are numbered 1 through 6. Assume that after vigorously stirring the applesauce, each micro-tablet could be anywhere in the applesauce. Then each tablet has a 50-50 chance of being in the half of the applesauce consumed on day 4. So each micro-tablet is like a fair coin that comes up either head (consumed on day 4) or tail (consumed on day 5). In essence, the population G of interest consists of all possible head-tail sequences of six coin tosses, with all sequences equally likely. The event E of interest is the subset of such sequences with exactly three heads. It can be shown that $P(E) = 20/64$, which is about 31%.

What is the probability of getting the recommended two micro-tablets on each of the days 1, 2, 3? Only about 12%! It's more complicated to obtain this number than it was for days 4 and 5, but a similar approach does the job.

So, if the goal is to avoid over-dosing or under-dosing in the first five days, then the instruction to dilute capsules in applesauce is clearly not the best way to go.

Example 7. A dog of a different color: Most people know the Doberman Pinscher in its black form (black with tan markings), but it also has red, blue, and fawn color forms. The four coat colors are controlled by two genes, *black* and *dilute*, each having a dominant and recessive allele. Let B and D stand for the black-dominant and dilute-dominant alleles, and let b and d stand for the corresponding recessive alleles. Let $B\blacklozenge$ stand for either allele pair BB or Bb, and let $D\blacklozenge$ stand for either allele pair DD or Dd. Here's how Doberman color is determined when the parents each contribute an allele for black and an allele for dilute: Black $B\blacklozenge D\blacklozenge$; Red $bbD\blacklozenge$; Blue $B\blacklozenge dd$; and Fawn $bbdd$.

What is the probability that two parent dogs, both heterozygous for black and dilute (i.e., both of genotype $BbDd$), will conceive a fawn pup? It's as though each parent dog tosses two fair coins, one called *black* with faces B and b, and the other called *dilute* with faces D and d. We are asking for the probability that both dogs toss the pair (b, d). The probability of that happening is $1/2^4$, which is $1/16$. This approach works for other parents and other pups.

Interestingly, it has been observed that Doberman coat color is correlated with the disease profile of the animal. However, the genetic underpinnings of Doberman color are simple compared to the genetic basis for some human diseases like autism, breast cancer, coronary disease, and many others. Dozens of genes acting alone or in concert have been implicated in these diseases. Analyzing this information and tapping it for diagnosis and treatment is far more challenging, and goes far beyond what humans can do. Without the computer, it's hopeless.

Example 8. Heart trouble: What is the probability that a man who is fifty years old will at some point in the future experience a first heart attack? We might try to answer this question by looking at some historical data, taking the population G to be the set of all male patients in a database who died after age fifty from any cause, but were heart-attack-free at age fifty. The event E of interest is the subset of those patients who experienced a heart attack after age fifty. The fraction of such patients is $n(E)/n(G)$.

A man, presently at age fifty and heart-attack-free, might be viewed as similar to any of the patients in the population G, so that his future experience regarding heart attack might be like taking a random draw from G, where all members of G are equally likely. From this perspective, the man's probability of getting a heart attack is the probability of the event E, which is $P(E) = n(E)/n(G)$.

How reliable is this estimate of his heart attack risk? The answer depends on how the database was assembled and the number of patients in the database. We will take up this kind of question in Chapter 9.

Example 9. Pink or blue, girl or boy? Some over-the-counter do-it-at-home tests claim to give you the gender of the baby at seven weeks of pregnancy with 95% accuracy, that accuracy improving as the term increases.

Such a test can have ethical implications: If genetic screening of the parents suggests a high risk for a severe gender-dependent medical condition in the offspring (e.g., hemophilia or fragile X syndrome), then the parents may choose to terminate the pregnancy if the test suggests the fetus has the high-risk gender. Setting aside the debate of pro-choice vs. pro-life, such termination would be especially unfortunate if the test result was incorrect. Can we trust the manufacturer's claim that the test is 95% accurate?

In order to sell the test on the market, the FDA required the manufacturer to perform a clinical trial on a sample of pregnant women – a small subset of the larger population of pregnant women. On the sample, the test may indeed have been 95% accurate. But how accurate is it on the larger population? How confident can we be that the test performance is within, say, 1% of the claimed 95%, when considering the larger population? Without more information, not very confident! We'll have much more to say about this in Chapter 9.

Probability when outcomes are not equally likely

Not everything that counts can be counted; and not everything that can be counted counts.

Albert Einstein

In all of the examples above, the outcomes in the finite population G were equally likely. In this case the correct way to compute the probability of an event E in G is to use probability by counting, which sets $P(E)$ equal to $n(E)/n(G)$.

On the other hand, if the outcomes in G are not equally likely, but have known probabilities, then the appropriate way to compute the probability $P(E)$ of an event E is to sum the probabilities of the outcomes in E.

What if you apply this latter method to a finite population

whose outcomes *are* equally likely? You get the same answer as probability by counting. (If all the outcomes in G are equally likely, then the probability of each outcome is $1/n(G)$, and the probability of an event E in G is $n(E)$ times $1/n(G)$, which equals $n(E)/n(G)$ – same answer as probability by counting.)

Example 10. Tossing a loaded die: A loaded die has the same faces as a fair die, so again $G = \{1, 2, 3, 4, 5, 6\}$, but the probabilities of those faces are not necessarily the same. Suppose the face probabilities are: $P(\{1\}) = P(\{2\}) = 2/20$, $P(\{3\}) = 7/20$, and $P(\{4\}) = P(\{5\}) = P(\{6\}) = 3/20$. What is the probability of the event of tossing a 2, 3 or 5? Here E is the event $\{2, 3, 5\}$ and it occurs with probability $P(E) = 2/20 + 7/20 + 3/20 = 12/20$, which equals 3/5.

Example 11. Blood type: There are four primary blood types: A, B, AB, and O. Take the population of outcomes G to be the set $\{A, B, AB, O\}$. As it happens, about 42% of US citizens are of type A, 10% of type B, 4% of type AB, and 44% of type O. What is the probability that a randomly selected person in the US has blood type A or B? This is equivalent to selecting a random outcome in G, which is governed by the indicated probabilities. The event E of interest is $\{A, B\}$, and the probability $P(E)$ of this event is $P(\{A\}) + P(\{B\}) = 42\% + 10\% = 52\%$.

Probability on infinite populations

The following examples show how to compute the probability of an event when the population of outcomes G is infinite.

Example 12. Probability as area, volume, and length: Suppose G is a region of finite area painted on the floor. Though G has finite area, if viewed as a population of points, it contains infinitely many points. Suppose E is a sub-region (event) within G. What is the probability that the next cosmic ray from outer space that hits G also hits E? The cosmic ray can be reasonably viewed as picking a point from G at random, with all points in G

equally likely. Within G, the probability $P(E)$ that the cosmic ray hits a point in E is reasonably defined as the area of E divided by the area of G.

Suppose that G is a finite volume of space and E is a sub-volume of G. If we pick a random point in G, then the probability $P(E)$ that the selected point belongs to E is sensibly defined as the volume of E divided by the volume of G. Suppose G is a line and E is subset of this line. If we pick a random point in G, then the probability $P(E)$ that that point belongs to E is sensibly defined as length of E divided by length of G.

Example 13. Probability as area under a curve: Here's an example that involves what's called a *bell curve* (alternatively, a *Normal distribution curve*). An instance of such a curve is shown in Figure 7-1 representing the distribution of IQ scores among all US citizens. The horizontal axis is IQ. The total area between the curve and the horizontal axis is assumed to be one. Here's how the curve can be used: If E is any subset of IQ's – say for example, the interval from 115 to 130 – then the *fraction* of US citizens

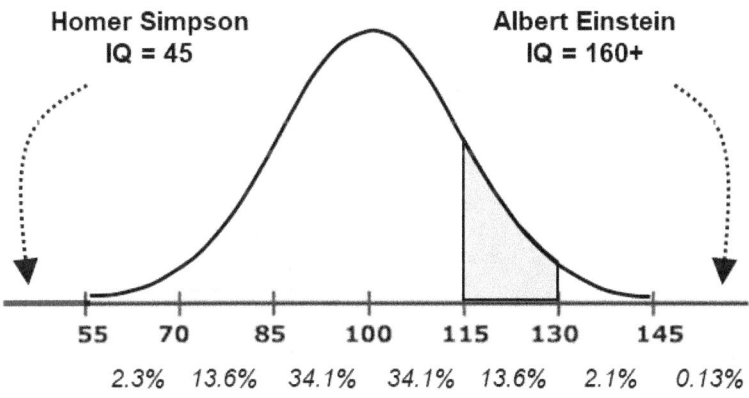

Figure 7-1 *The bell curve representing the distribution of IQ scores across all US citizens. The total area under the curve is taken to be one. The event E is the interval from 115 to 130 along the horizontal IQ-axis. The probability P(E) assigned to event E by the bell curve is the area of the gray region shown, which is about 13.6%.*

having IQ in the interval E is well-approximated by the area of the gray region above E and below the curve. In this case, the area is 13.6%.

Let's look at things another way: Let G be the population of possible IQ's, as represented by the IQ-axis. We can view the interval E from 115 to 130 as an event in G. Define the probability $P(E)$ of event E as the area of the gray region above E and below the curve. What is the *probability* that a person selected at random from among all US citizens has IQ in the interval E? The answer is well-approximated by $P(E)$. In this case, 13.6%.

In general, any curve above the horizontal x-axis (for some measurement x) having total area one between itself and the x-axis is called a **probability distribution curve**. Figure 7-2 shows a probability distribution curve that is decidedly not bell-shaped. This curve may represent the distribution of x-values measured across a large group of individuals. As before, take G to be the x-axis, and E to be any subset (event) in G. Define $P(E)$ to be the area of the gray region between E and the curve, as shown in the figure. If an individual is selected from the group at random, then $P(E)$ is the approximate probability that the individual's x-value is within E.

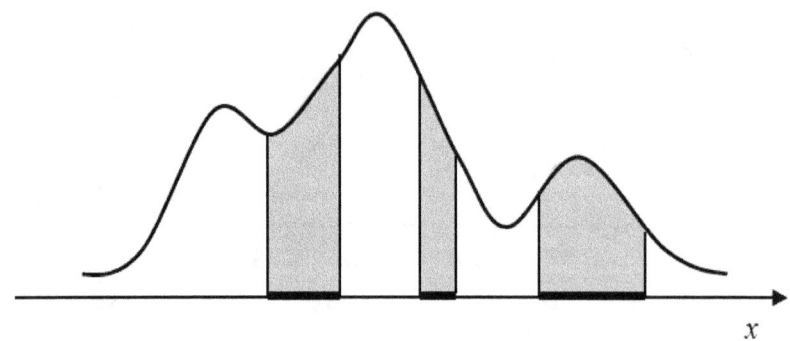

Figure 7-2 *A probability distribution curve above the x-axis having total area one between itself and the x-axis. A subset (event) E of the x-axis is shown and consists of three disjoint intervals. The probability P(E) assigned to event E by the distribution curve is the area of the gray region.*

Example 14: Probability as volume under a surface. Just as area under a curve can be viewed as associating probabilities with subsets (events) of the horizontal *x*-axis, volume under a surface can be viewed as associating probabilities with subsets (events) of the horizontal *xy*-plane. Suppose we have a surface representing the distribution of measurement pairs (x, y) across all US citizens, where x is, say, body height, and y is body weight. Figure 7-3 shows a contrived example of such a surface. Assume the total volume under the surface is one. Let E be any subset of the *xy*-plane, say for example, the gray rectangle shown in the figure. Then the fraction of US citizens whose measurement pairs (x, y) are contained within E is well-approximated by the volume above E and below the surface.

Here's another way to look at it: Take G to be the *xy*-plane and view E as an event in G. Define the probability $P(E)$ to be the volume just described. If a person is selected at random from

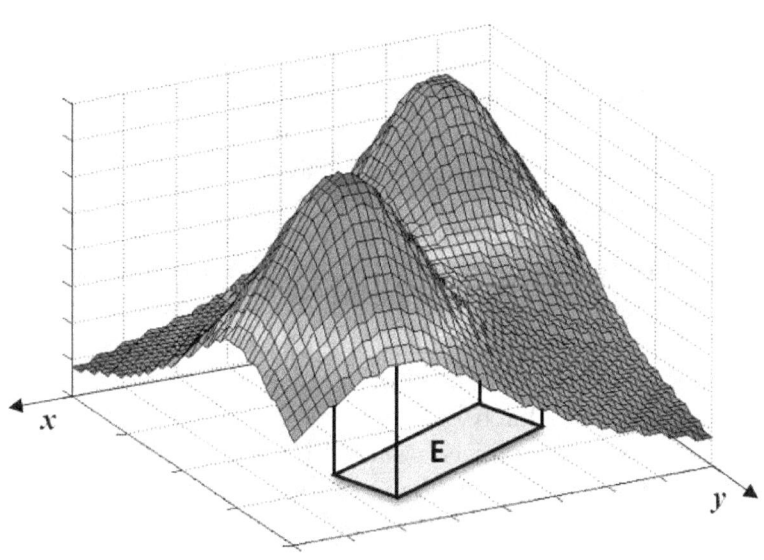

Figure 7-3 *A probability distribution surface above the xy-plane having total volume one between itself and the xy-plane. A subset (event) E of the xy-plane is shown (in general it need not be a rectangle). The probability P(E) assigned to event E by the distribution surface is the volume between E and the surface.*

among all US citizens, then $P(E)$ is the approximate probability that the person's measurement pair (x, y) is contained within E.

Of course, there may be more than two measurements for a particular application. In this case we have to think more abstractly. Depicting surfaces and volumes in dimensions greater than three is not possible, but the mathematics for computing $P(E)$ remains essentially the same as it is for smaller dimensions. Mathematics gives us the information we need, regardless of whether we can picture the object or not. That's the power of abstraction, the power of mathematics.

Probability histograms

A **probability histogram** is a diagram showing the fraction of individuals in a group who fall into discrete categories. The categories are assumed to be *exclusive* (no individual belongs to more than one category) and *exhaustive* (every individual belongs to some category). The categories may be derived from disjoint intervals of a numerical measurement (e.g., disjoint intervals of age or blood pressure) or correspond to the possible values of a discrete characteristic (e.g., race or profession).

Figure 7-4 is an example of a probability histogram. The group consists of women in a study all of whom were diagnosed with breast cancer. In this example, the measurement is the age at which the diagnosis occurred. The age axis has been divided into intervals (categories) that are a decade wide. Each interval is referred to as a **bin**. Each bin supports a rectangular **bar**. The total area of the histogram is assumed to be one. The area of a bar indicates the fraction of women in the group who reside in the corresponding bin. (Note: If all the bins have the same width, and that width is considered to be one unit, then the height of a bar and the area of a bar are identical.) If we were to pick an individual at random from the group, then the area of a bar indicates the probability that the individual was selected from the corresponding bin.

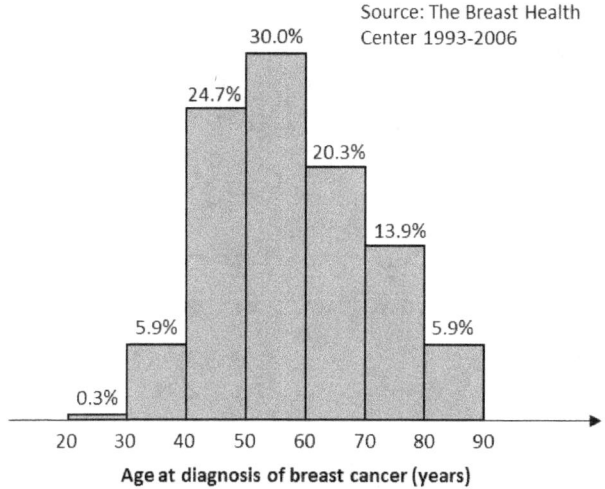

Figure 7-4 *In a study of women who were diagnosed with breast cancer, the probability histogram indicates, for each decade of life, the fraction of women in the study who received the diagnosis in that decade. The total area of the histogram is one. The area of each bar is indicated.*

Another way of indicating the fraction of individuals who fall into each category is with a **pie chart**, like the one shown in Figure 7-5. The total area of the pie is assumed to be one. The area of each sector is the fraction of individuals in the associated category.

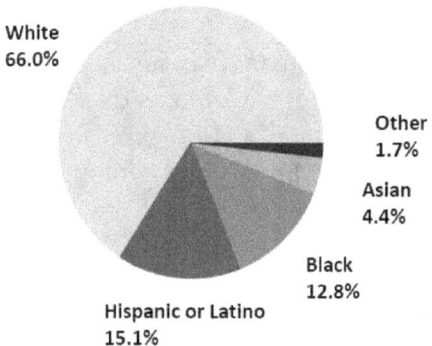

Figure 7-5 *A pie chart based on the 2009 US census showing the fraction of US persons by race at that time. The total area of the pie is one. The area of each sector is indicated.*

In some applications, two measurements, x and y, are each assessed on the individuals in a group, where, x might be, say, body height, and y might be body weight. A *3D probability histogram* indicates the fraction of individuals in the group who fall into distinct categories, where now the categories correspond to rectangular cells in the xy-plane. See Figure 7-6. Here each cell is a bin that supports a parallelepiped bar. The total volume of the histogram is assumed to be one. The volume of a bar indicates the fraction of individuals in the group who fall into the corresponding bin.

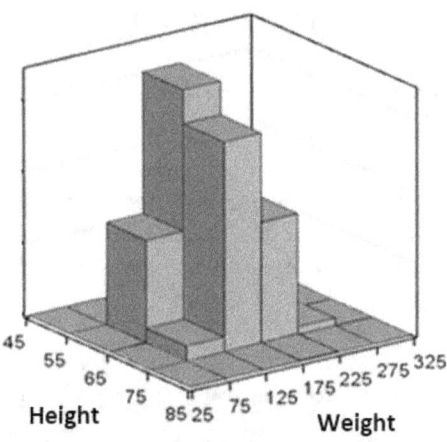

Figure 7-6 *A 3D probability histogram for body height and body weight in a group of individuals. The total volume of the histogram is one.*

When there are more than two measurements, we cannot depict the associated higher-dimensional histograms, but discussing them mathematically is no problem – the abstraction of mathematics handles all dimensions with equal facility.

Other bar charts

A probability histogram is a special kind of **bar chart** in which the areas (volumes) of the bars sum to one. In other bar charts, we don't care about the areas (volumes) of the bars, but rather their heights, and there is no restriction on these heights – they don't have to sum to one. In many bar charts, the categories are still exclusive and exhaustive, but that's not true of others.

Often a bar chart is constructed as follows: Take two measurements, x and y, on all the individuals in a group. Next, partition the individuals into bins corresponding to disjoint intervals of the x-measurement. Then for each bin, compute the average y-value of the individuals in that bin, and stand up a rectangular bar whose height is that average y-value. Label the horizontal axis x and the vertical axis y.

Figure 7-7 shows a bar chart for a group of US citizens, where the x-measurement is age, and the y-measurement is Body Mass Index (BMI), defined as body weight (in kilograms) divided by the square of body height (in meters).

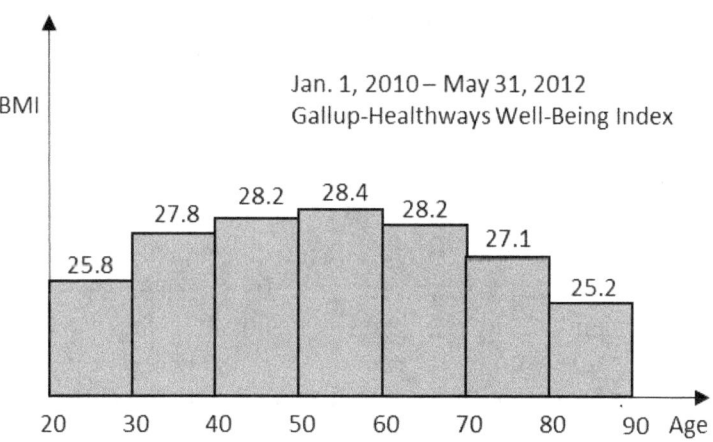

Figure 7-7 *A bar chart indicating average BMI by decade of age in a group of US citizens. The height of each bar is indicated.*

Figure 7-8 shows a bar chart for a group of US men, where the x-measurement is age, and the y-measurement is 0 or 1, depending on whether or not the individual shows symptoms of coronary heart disease: 1 = yes; 0 = no. In this case, the average *y*-value of a bin equals the *fraction* of individuals in the bin who have coronary heart disease.

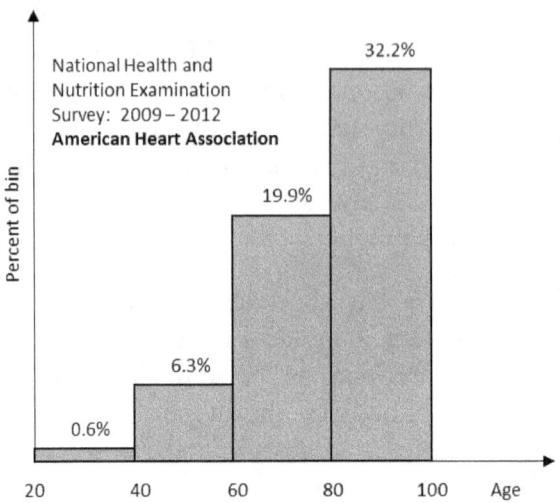

Figure 7-8 *A bar chart indicating the fraction of US men in each twenty-year period who have coronary heart disease. The height of each bar is indicated.*

The categories (bins) in some bar charts might not necessarily be exclusive (an individual might belong to more than one category.) For example, you might have a bar chart where the categories are labeled with the possible side effects from a drug, and the height of a bar indicates the fraction of patients in a study who experienced the associated side effect. In this case, a patient could be present in more than one category.

Of course, just as for histograms, there can be three-dimensional bar charts and higher-dimensional bar charts.

Over-binning

On television and in print, you often see ads claiming that some new pharmaceutical will greatly improve life by promoting better sleep, increased vigor, enhanced appearance, or making a more vibrant and sexier you. The ads often feature ordinary people, supposedly like the rest of us, but extraordinarily good-looking, without any age blemishes. They're jogging, dancing, or cavorting in bed – clearly living life to the fullest. This is then followed by a seemingly endless list of possible side-effects that in some cases occupies the bulk of the commercial.

Why does Big Pharma do this? To convey the message: "You can trust us. Look how honest and open we are. Yes, we're telling you that there are risks of side effects – small risks really – but we have your health and safety in mind, and just want you to be fully informed." Sure, this protects Big Pharma from charges that they did not exercise due diligence in alerting consumers to possible risks. But by "binning" (characterizing) the side effects so narrowly, the message to the audience is that the risks are rare and of little concern.

Instead, it would be more helpful to consumers if the stated side effects were logically grouped together using far fewer bins. For example, decreased resistance to cold, flu, and pneumonia, or increased susceptibility to arthritis flare-ups, eczema, and psoriasis, could be considered six distinct side effects of a particular drug. But it would be more useful to recognize all of them as possible manifestations of a compromised immune system.

Is over-binning Big Pharma's way of "hiding the forest behind the trees"?

What exactly is probability?

In the examples of this chapter, we saw different ways of assigning probability to the events of a population without saying what probability *actually* is. Though all of us have some vague, intuitive notions about it, probability is a tricky concept to define: What does it really mean to say that a "coin is fair", that "the probability of tossing heads is 50%"? What does it really mean to say "draw a marble at random from a hat, with all marbles equally likely"?

Because probability is such a slippery notion, we will avoid trying to say what it is, and shift our focus instead to identifying rules about how it behaves; then look for the logical consequences of those rules. This kind of approach is not uncommon in science. Isaac Newton posited his Universal Law of Gravitation in 1687, which describes how gravity behaves – but what gravity is was a total mystery in his time. (Today, from Einstein, we know that gravity can be viewed as a bending of space-time, and from the recent LIGO experiment, that gravity can propagate as a wave.)

The study of probability originated in the 1650's motivated by questions from gambling. Later, many other applications emerged: in census-taking, insurance, physics, and other areas. For a long time, probability questions were answered in an ad hoc manner. Then in 1933, Andrey Kolmogorov came up with three simple properties that any **probability measure** should satisfy. A probability measure P refers to any method for assigning likelihoods to the events in a population. Which measure to use for a given application depends on the application, and is usually driven by the need for a mathematical model that adequately characterizes a real-world behavior involving chance.

Kolmogorov's Axioms of Probability:

- *$0 \leq P(E) \leq 1$, for any event E*
- *$P(G) = 1$, where G is the population*
- *$P(E \cup F) = P(E) + P(F)$ for any events E and F having no members in common (i.e., disjoint events)*

In other words, a probability measure on a population G has to satisfy three things: The probability of any event E (subset of G) is always a number between zero and one; the probability of the event *G* itself is one; and the probability of the union of two disjoint events *E* and *F* is the probability of *E* plus the probability of *F*. (Note: The third bullet of the *official* Kolmogorov Axioms extends to "infinite unions of disjoint events", but that difference need not concern us here.)

Everyone agrees that these are true statements about how probability behaves. And amazingly, everything we know about probability can be logically derived from these three statements! Recalling Einstein: *Everything should be as simple as possible, but no simpler.*

Probability Theory refers to the set of logical consequences of the above axioms. The axioms are simple enough, yes, but some of their consequences take us well beyond our intuitions. The theory is very useful for telling us how to make correct probability calculations in a wide variety of settings including medicine, and for telling us what can and cannot be reasonably inferred from empirical data. We'll encounter some of this theory in the following chapters.

Abstraction is the mother of generalization, and the abstraction resulting from the Kolmogorov Axioms allows you to analyze coin tossing experiments and drug efficacy trials from the same point of view, making use of the same mathematical framework.

A probability measure is sometimes called a **probability distribution**. Again, it refers to any method for assigning probabilities to the events (subsets) of a population, where the method satisfies the Kolmogorov Axioms. For example, on a finite population, probability by counting is a probability distribution – one in which all the outcomes (singleton events) have equal probability. A probability histogram is a probability distribution: the population is the set of bins; the probability of a bin is the area of its corresponding bar; an event is a subset of bins; and the probability of the event is the sum of the bar areas for those bins. A probability distribution curve is a probability distribution: the population is the set of (infinitely many) points along the horizontal axis; an event is a subset of those points; and the probability of the event is the area between the subset and the curve.

Ch. 8 Conditional Probability and Bayes' Formula

Probability depends on the population you're looking at. What is the probability of developing breast cancer? Among women it's one thing; among men it's something else. What's the probability of developing lung cancer? Are we talking about smokers or non-smokers? And so it goes with all probability statements. We need to know what population is being referred to in order for a probability to have meaning.

Sometimes a probability question about an initial population will have its focus narrowed to a subpopulation. For example, maybe the original population consists of all people in the US, and we're asking: What is the probability that a randomly chosen person from this population has a certain disease D? (This is the same as asking, what is the **prevalence** of the disease in the population, i.e., the fraction of the population who have the disease?) Suppose a diagnostic test T is available for detecting the disease, but the test is not perfect. We might ask: What is the probability that a randomly chosen person who shows test positive actually has the disease? (Equivalently, what is the prevalence of the disease among people who are test positive?)

Let G denote the US population. To economize on notation,

we'll assign double-duty to the symbols D and T: Let D denote not only the disease, but also the subset of G consisting of all people who have the disease (are disease positive). Let T denote not only the test, but also the subset of G consisting of all people who would test positive for the disease if they were given the test. These subsets of G can be represented by what's called a *Venn diagram*. In such a diagram, the population G itself is usually represented as a rectangle, and the subsets of interest are usually represented as disks inside the rectangle. The radii of the disks are generally taken to be equal, but have no significance. What is important is whether or not the disks overlap. When two or more disks overlap, it means that their associated subsets of G may have elements in common.

Figure 8-1 shows some Venn diagrams with particular regions of interest highlighted in grey.

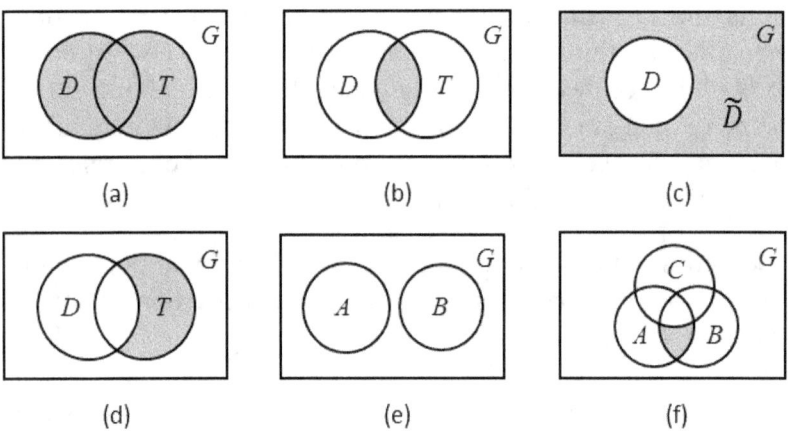

Figure 8-1 *Venn diagrams.*

In Figure 8-1(a), the grey region represents the *union* of D and T, denoted $D \cup T$, the subset of G whose members belong to D or T or both. In other words, it is the set of people in G who have the disease or would test positive for the disease or both.

In Figure 8-1(b), the grey region represents the *intersection* of D and T, denoted $D \cap T$, the subset of G whose members belong to both D and T. This is the set of people in G who have the disease and would test positive for it.

In Figure 8-1(c), the grey region represents the *complement* of D, denoted $\tilde{D}$, the subset of G whose members lie outside D. It is the set of people in G who do not have the disease.

In Figure 8-1(d), the grey region represents the *difference T minus D*, denoted $T \sim D$, which is another way of expressing the subset $T \cap \tilde{D}$, the subset of G whose members belong to T but not D. This set consists of all people in G who would test positive for the disease but do not actually have the disease. It is called the set of *false positives*. Similarly, the subset $D \sim T$ (not shown), which is another way of expressing $\tilde{T} \cap D$, consists of all people in G who would test negative for the disease even though they have the disease. It is called the set of *false negatives*.

Figure 8-1(e), which has no grey region, shows two subsets A and B with no members in common, and are called **disjoint**.

Finally, in Figure 8-1(f), three subsets A, B, and C are shown, and the grey region represents $(A \cap B) \cap \tilde{C}$, the subset of G whose members lie in A and B, but not in C.

The following probability relationships can be derived from the Kolmogorov axioms (and appreciated pictorially with Venn diagrams):

- $P(\tilde{D}) = 1 - P(D)$
- $P(D \cup T) = P(D) + P(T) - P(D \cap T) \leq P(D) + P(T)$
- $P(D \cap T) \geq 1 - P(\tilde{D}) - P(\tilde{T})$

Conditional probability

Often a probability question takes the form: "What is the probability of this *given* that?" For example, if a fair die is rolled, what is the probability of rolling a 5 given that the roll comes up odd? The probability of rolling a 5 is 1/6. But the probability of rolling a 5 given that the roll comes up odd is 1/3. Here's another example: What is the probability that a randomly chosen person in the US will develop lung cancer at some point in life given that the person smoked a pack a day for at least a decade?

In general, for any two events A and B in a population G, we denote the **conditional probability of A given B**, by the symbol $P(A|B)$. Using probability by counting, we define

$$P(A|B) = \frac{n(A \cap B)}{n(B)}.$$

Dividing numerator and denominator by $n(G)$, we see that

$$P(A|B) = \frac{P(A \cap B)}{P(B)}.$$

We take this as the definition of conditional probability (even when it's not probability by counting). The above definition leads to the following useful relationship:

$$P(A \cap B) = P(A|B) \times P(B).$$

Convention often dispenses with the explicit symbol "×" for multiplication, so that we can write (with the multiplication understood)

$$P(A \cap B) = P(A|B)P(B).$$

Without going into details, the definition of conditional probability satisfies the Kolmogorov Axioms. So any statement about probability that can be derived from the axioms also holds true for conditional probability. For example, it can be shown that for any pair of events E and B, we have $P(\widetilde{E}|B) = 1 - P(E|B)$. And for any pair of disjoint events E and F, we have $P((E \cup F)|B) = P(E|B) + P(F|B)$.

If D is the subset of individuals in a population G who have a particular disease (i.e., the event "disease positive"), and T is the subset of individuals in G who would test positive for the disease (i.e., the event "test positive"), then the following conditional probabilities listed with their common names are frequently of medical interest:

$P(T|\widetilde{D})$ – **false positive rate** of the test
$P(\widetilde{T}|D)$ – **false negative rate** of the test
$P(T|D)$ – **sensitivity** or **true positive rate** of the test
$P(\widetilde{T}|\widetilde{D})$ – **specificity** or **true negative rate** of the test
$P(D|T)$ – **positive prediction value** of the test
$P(\widetilde{D}|\widetilde{T})$ – **negative prediction value** of the test

A test T is considered at least somewhat useful in detecting disease D if the sensitivity (true positive rate) is greater than the false positive rate. (This relationship implies that $P(D|T) > P(D)$ and $P(\widetilde{D}|T) < P(\widetilde{D})$. It also implies that $P(\widetilde{D}|\widetilde{T}) > P(\widetilde{D})$ and that $P(D|\widetilde{T}) < P(D)$. It does not imply that $P(D|T) > 50\%$.)

The **false positive probability** of the test T is $P(T \cap \widetilde{D})$, which equals the false positive rate times $P(\widetilde{D})$. The **false negative probability** of the test T is $P(\widetilde{T} \cap D)$, which equals the false negative rate times $P(D)$. Similar formulas hold for the true positive and true negative probabilities.

The **total error probability** of the test T is the fraction of the population that is false positive or false negative, that is to say, it is the fraction, $P(T \cap \widetilde{D}) + P(\widetilde{T} \cap D)$. If the penalty value for a false positive is different from that for a false negative, then the total error probability is not a good measure of the quality of the test. In that case, it is more appropriate to use **total weighted error**, $[a \times P(T \cap \widetilde{D})] + [b \times P(\widetilde{T} \cap D)]$, where a is the amount of penalty associated with a false positive, and b is the amount of penalty associated with a false negative.

Conditional probability and the anti-vax activists

As reported in the article, "Why the Anti-Vaccine Crowd Won't Fade Away", *Time*, October 6, 2014, mumps vaccination is 80% to 90% effective, that is to say, $P(D|V)$ is 10-20% of $P(D|\tilde{V})$, where D is the subset of the population that gets the disease (mumps in this case), and V is the subset of the population that has been vaccinated. Not bad, but it could be better.

The same article reports a favorite argument of the anti-vax (anti-vaccination) crowd (quote): *...97% of the people who contract mumps have been vaccinated – so what is the point of getting the shot in the first place?* In other words, they point out that $P(V|D)$ is 97% and take that as justification for not getting the vaccine.

That's a big misunderstanding of conditional probability! It's not $P(V|D)$ that we're interested in, but rather $P(D|V)$ and how it compares with $P(D|\tilde{V})$. That $P(V|D)$ is so high in the US is a reflection of the high rate of vaccination in this country. To bring the mistake into stark relief, imagine a community where *everyone* gets vaccinated for a certain disease D. Then if even just one person comes down with the disease, we must conclude that $P(V|D)$ is 100% – but to use that as justification not to vaccinate makes no sense!

If enough people are persuaded by the anti-vax message, then many diseases that are on the verge of extinction will be given a reprieve (e.g., polio, whooping cough, measles, and many more).

In the article, "Anti-vaccine activists spark US state's worst measles outbreak in decades", *Washington Post*, May 5, 2017, it is stated that (quote): *The vaccination rate for measles, mumps, and rubella began falling sharply a decade ago among children of Somali descent who live in Minnesota. That drop is now being blamed for a major measles outbreak within the Somali American community there.* Measles can kill. Unfortunately, this community fell under the spell of influential anti-vax activists, like fraudster-in-chief Dr. Andrew Wakefield.

And it's not enough that just some or most of us get vaccinated. In order to achieve *herd immunity*, which prevents a disease from spreading rapidly throughout the herd, a high proportion of the individuals must be vaccinated.

Independent events

Two nonempty events E and F in a population are said to be **independent** if the occurrence of F does not affect the probability of E, and vice versa. In symbols, E and F are said to be independent if $P(E|F) = P(E)$, or equivalently, $P(F|E) = P(F)$. More succinctly, using the definition of conditional probability, E and F are said to be independent if $P(E \cap F) = P(E)P(F)$, that is, $P(E \cap F)$ equals $P(E)$ times $P(F)$. If E and F are independent, then it can be shown that E and $\tilde{F}$ are also independent, and similarly, $\tilde{E}$ and $\tilde{F}$ are independent.

A word of caution – don't confuse *independent* events with *disjoint* events: If E and F are nonempty disjoint events, then the event $E \cap F$ is empty, meaning that $P(E \cap F)$ is zero; if E and F are nonempty independent events, then $P(E \cap F) = P(E)P(F)$, which is nonzero.

Two events E and F that are not independent are said to be **dependent.** Dependence and independence are important concepts in medicine. You might want to know, for example, if having a certain medical condition increases the likelihood of having some other medical condition. For example, obesity and diabetes are dependent. But flat feet and astigmatism are independent (we guess).

Let's look at a couple more examples:

Toss two fair dice, one red and one blue. Let G be the population of all possible outcome pairs (r, b), where r is the value of the red die, and b is the value of the blue die. The total numbers of pairs in G is $6 \times 6 = 36$, all pairs equally likely.

Let E be the event that the red die comes up 1 or 2. Let F be the event that the blue die comes up 2, 3, or 4. Then E and F are independent: There are 6 out of 36 pairs (r, b) that satisfy both events simultaneously, so $P(E \cap F) = 6/36 = 1/6$. But also, 12 out of 36 pairs satisfy event E alone, and 18 out of 36 pairs satisfy event F alone. So $P(E) = 12/36 = 1/3$ and $P(F) = 18/36 = 1/2$, which means $P(E)P(F) = (1/3)(1/2) = 1/6 = P(E \cap F)$. In this example, the fact that E and F are independent events comes as no surprise – the outcome of the red die clearly has no bearing on the outcome of the blue die, and vice versa.

Let E_6 be the event that the sum of the two dice is 6. Let E_7 be the event that their sum is 7. And let F be the event that the red die comes up 4. Then $P(E_6|F) = 1/6$ and $P(E_6) = 5/36$. So $P(E_6|F) \neq P(E_6)$ and thus E_6 and F are dependent. On the other hand, $P(E_7|F) = 1/6$ while $P(E_7) = 6/36 = 1/6$. So E_7 and F are independent. This example shows that it's not always obvious at the outset whether two events are independent. Sometimes we have to do a little math to find out.

Given two events in a population, we might ask: How much dependence is there between them? Such a measure is called a *correlation*, and there are many different ways to define it. Which one to use depends on the application.

If two events are correlated (i.e., dependent), then knowing that one event has occurred increases or decreases the probability of the other event occurring. But be careful – *correlation does not imply causation*: Heavy smoking and drinking have significant correlation, but neither is a cause of the other. Instead, both may be a reflection of a third *confounding factor*: a person who is generally prone to addictive behaviors.

The ideal sample

Suppose you want to determine the prevalence $P(D)$ of a disease in a population G. But if G is very large or not fully accessible, then a complete survey of all its members is impractical. In that case, here's what is done: Get a small "representative" sample F from the population G, and use the prevalence in F to estimate the prevalence in G. In other words, you take $P(D|F)$ as an approximation to $P(D)$.

An ideal sample F for this purpose is one in which the subsets (events) D and F are independent, because then $P(D) = P(D|F)$. Unfortunately, there is no assured way of getting a hold of an ideal sample. But what we can do is select members of G at random to participate in the sample F, and cross our fingers that the resulting sample is nearly independent of D. It turns out that this becomes increasingly likely as the sample size increases – which lends credence to the whole statistical (sample-based) approach to understanding the world. We'll be more quantitative about this in Chapter 9.

The statistical approach is used to assess the sensitivity and specificity of tests, their false negative and false positive rates, and prediction values. It's used in FDA clinical trials to assess efficacy and safety of new drugs. It's used in other studies to assess efficacy and safety of devices, and surgical procedures. It's used extensively in science, marketing, political polling, public health, and many other areas.

The elusive gold standard

For us, a **gold standard** test for a disease or condition is a test which either: (a) serves as the very definition of the disease or (b) has no false positives or false negatives relative to an independent established definition of the disease. The notion of gold standard is a somewhat slippery concept. Certain diseases and conditions have a universally accepted gold standard (e.g., broken bone, arsenic poisoning, polio, Ebola); others do not (e.g., high blood pressure, unhealthy liver function, fibromyalgia, autism, among many others).

Even if a disease or condition has a gold standard, the test might not always be *practical* to administer: it might require post-mortem analysis, or might be too expensive, too inconvenient, too painful, or not timely enough. So the medical community is always in pursuit of the best practical test for a disease – a test that is practical to administer and as close as possible to being a gold standard.

Here are some examples of diseases that have a gold standard, but presently do not have a practical gold standard: Alzheimer's disease, life-threatening prostate cancer, life-threatening breast cancer, and life-threatening kidney disease. The present gold standard for Alzheimer's disease requires a post-mortem analysis of brain tissue. The present gold standards for life-threatening prostate cancer and life-threating breast cancer require waiting until it's clear that the patient will succumb to the cancer unless there's a medical intervention. Similarly, the gold standard for life-threatening kidney disease is the observation of kidney failure or some other dangerous consequence of lowered kidney function. Unfortunately, all practical existing tests for these diseases have high false positive rates. Regarding prostate cancer and breast cancer, these tests have resulted in high rates of over-treatment.

Another example of a disease with a gold standard, but not a very practical one, is Ebola: At least as recently as 2014, the gold standard test proceeded as follows. A person who is suspected of having Ebola is first placed in quarantine for up to 21 days, as that is how long it can take for the fever to show up, and the virus is not detectable in blood until after the fever arrives. With onset of fever, blood is extracted, prepared in cell culture, and then several days later, examined microscopically for evidence of the virus.

Clearly this gold standard is neither timely nor convenient. A 21-day quarantine represents quite an impact to a person's life, especially if the test comes back negative. Also, in some places, especially in third world countries, "quarantine" often means being placed in a makeshift ward with other patients. If you didn't have Ebola to begin with, you might well end up with it.

Today, there is a rapid antigen test for Ebola which gives

results in 15 minutes. It has a sensitivity of 92% and specificity of 85%. (See Wikipedia, "Ebola virus disease").

Bayes' Theorem

Probability often behaves in subtle, unintuitive, and even counterintuitive ways.

Here's an example. Suppose that 5% of the population G has a disease. Suppose that a test for the disease is 95% *accurate* in the following sense: 95% of persons who have the disease show test positive, and 95% of persons who don't have the disease show test negative. But now, what is the probability that a person who shows test positive has the disease? We'll see in a few moments that the answer is only 50% – on average only 50 out of 100 people who present a positive test actually have the disease! That's a real surprise to most people. Even faculty and students in medical schools often guess much higher, often somewhere in the range of 90% to 95%.

During the early days of the AIDS outbreak, the best test for the disease had roughly the same accuracy, 95%, and the AIDS disease itself had a prevalence that was in fact well below 5%.

To get the probability of disease positive given test positive, we need the renowned theorem of Thomas Bayes (1701 – 1761), an English mathematician and Presbyterian minister. Here's his theorem in all its generality and abstraction. Recall that D denotes the event of having the disease, and T denotes the event of testing positive for the disease.

***Bayes' Theorem (Formula)*:**

$$P(D|T) = \frac{P(T|D)P(D)}{P(T|D)P(D) + P(T|\widetilde{D})P(\widetilde{D})}$$

Let's see what happens when we apply this formula to our example above, where $P(T|D) = 0.95$, $P(T|\tilde{D}) = 1 - P(\tilde{T}|\tilde{D}) = 0.05$, $P(D) = 0.05$, and $P(\tilde{D}) = 0.95$. Substituting these values into Bayes Formula yields $P(D|T) = 50\%$, as claimed. The test is 95% accurate, yes, but half of those who would present a positive test do not have the disease! (By swapping symbols D and $\tilde{D}$ and symbols T and $\tilde{T}$ in Bayes' Formula above, we find that $P(\tilde{D}|\tilde{T}) = 99.7\%$, which is excellent. Evidently the test has low positive prediction value but high negative prediction value.)

So what does this mean? Are we talking about a lousy test? Not necessarily. For sure it has low positive prediction value, $P(D|T)$. The reason is that although the test is accurate, the disease has low prevalence $P(D)$ in the population G. If we were to restrict G to include only people at risk for the disease, perhaps those expressing early symptoms, or in the case of AIDS, those with a higher-risk lifestyle, then the disease prevalence will be greater in the new population, and so $P(D|T)$ will be much larger. (At the same time, this increase in prevalence will cause the negative prediction value $P(\tilde{D}|\tilde{T})$ to decrease.)

Many people find the practical implications of Bayes' Theorem so perplexing and counterintuitive that they are reluctant to accept them. But Bayes' Theorem is a theorem – a provable mathematical statement. Since the proof is so short and straightforward, we decided to present it here:

Recall the definition of conditional probability:

$$P(D|T) = \frac{P(D \cap T)}{P(T)}.$$

Since $P(D \cap T) = P(T \cap D) = P(T|D)P(D)$, we can rewrite the above as:

$$P(D|T) = \frac{P(T|D)P(D)}{P(T)} \quad (*)$$

Let's get another expression for $P(T)$. Since $T \cap D$ and $T \cap \tilde{D}$ are disjoint events whose union is T, we have:

$$P(T) = P(T \cap D) + P(T \cap \tilde{D}).$$

The two terms on the right can be rewritten as:

$$P(T) = P(T|D)P(D) + P(T|\tilde{D})P(\tilde{D}).$$

Plugging this back into the equation above labeled (*) gives us Bayes' Formula. Done!

Chapter 4 (section "Unregulated use of laboratory developed tests") discussed the FDA's concerns over marketed laboratory tests that make unfounded claims of accuracy. One such test claimed a positive prediction value of 99.3% in its ability to determine whether or not a woman would develop ovarian cancer. When the test was studied by independent biostatisticians not affiliated with the originating laboratory, they observed a positive prediction value of only 6.5%! The discrepancy occurred because the lab had constructed a study sample in which half the women were known to have ovarian cancer. That's far greater than the prevalence of ovarian cancer in the general population, and Bayes' Formula is sensitive to prevalence. (Again see, "Why the FDA Wants More Control over Some Lab Tests", *Scientific American*, Dec. 2016.)

Bayes' Formula is used commonly in practice because it enables us to estimate a probability that's "hard" to estimate directly by combining probabilities that are "easy" to estimate directly:

Without going into detail, trying to get a reliable estimate of $P(D|T)$ directly requires identifying a significant sub-sample of individuals who are T positive within a sample taken from the general population. If the disease is rare and T happens to be fairly accurate, then the latter sample – all of whose members will be subjected to test T – has to be large. This may not be practical. In other words, it may be "hard" to estimate $P(D|T)$

directly. By contrast, a reliable estimate of $P(T|D)$ can often be obtained from a much smaller sample consisting of individuals already known to have the disease. So $P(T|D)$ may be "easy" to estimate directly. Similarly, this is true for $P(T|\widetilde{D})$. Note that estimating $P(T|D)$ from a sample – estimating it as $n(T \cap D)/n(D)$ – does not require knowledge of the disease prevalence $P(D)$. And though we nevertheless do require an estimate of disease prevalence for Bayes' Formula, if the disease isn't new, an estimate of $P(D)$ may already exist from previous studies, and thus "easy" to obtain. Otherwise, a gold standard test has to be applied to a sample of the population, and that sample may have to be large if the disease is rare.

In the context of Bayes' Formula, $P(T|D)$ and $P(T|\widetilde{D})$ are called *prior probabilities* (since they indicate the extent to which the test result can be inferred from prior disease knowledge of the population), while $P(D|T)$ is called a *posterior probability* (since it indicates the extent to which disease knowledge of the population can be inferred from the test result).

In some medical applications, the population of interest consists not of two classes (D and $\widetilde{D}$), but rather three or more classes, each representing a distinct condition of the patient. For instance, suppose patients in the population have one of three conditions A, B, or C. Suppose there's a new diagnostic test available for deciding which of the three conditions the patient has. Understanding that the test may not be perfect, we may want to know: What is the probability that a patient has condition A given that the test result says the patient has condition A? Let T_A denote the event that the test result says condition A. Then we're interested in the conditional probability $P(A|T_A)$. The relevant version of Bayes' Formula is:

$$P(A|T_A) = \frac{P(T_A|A)P(A)}{P(T_A|A)P(A) + P(T_A|B)P(B) + P(T_A|C)P(C)}$$

Ch. 9 The Right Sample Size

During an election, while the voting booths are active, the media often makes predictions about district results. You might hear something like this: *With 8% of the ballots in, we are 95% certain that Branford Bogus will take 57% of the district, plus or minus 2%.* And far more often than not, they're right. How do they do that? Is it luck? Intuition? A crystal ball? No! – It's just sound mathematics (probability and statistics) – the kind of stuff covered in this chapter.

By contrast, when the media reports on medical matters – diseases, medications, and treatments – the numbers conveyed to the public are less detailed than for elections. You'll hear statements like "women with the *BRCA1* mutation have an 84% risk of breast cancer," or "the prevalence of adult HIV in South Africa is 17%," or "this new drug is 75% effective in treating such-and-such condition", without mentioning the "accuracy and confidence" (to be defined later) that should go along with these numbers, that is to say, without mentioning their reliability.

When studying a population that is large or not fully accessible, a researcher will try to extract a "representative" sample from the population and then use the results from that sample to estimate what's going on in the population as a whole. That said, there is no way to validate that a sample is representative. However, to the extent that the method of selecting the sample is unbiased, the sample may be regarded as "randomly" chosen from the population, and the hope is that this implies the sample is representative of the population. Such thought process is what underlies the statistical-empirical approach to gaining knowledge of the world.

In this chapter, we'll see that the above strategy is well-justified. We'll see that the larger a random sample, the more likely it is to be representative, and hence the more likely it is to be a good predictor of the larger population. But a larger sample typically equates to more time, money, and effort for collection and analysis. Is there reason to believe that sampling can be both reliable and practical? Yes! In fact, remarkably small random samples can make predictions with a surprising degree of accuracy and confidence. For instance, a random sample of size of 384 is already sufficient to estimate the prevalence of a disease to within 5% accuracy at 95% confidence, no matter what the population size. We'll soon explain the meaning of that statement.

But before we get into that, we need to recall, and beef-up our everyday notion of average, as well as introduce the concept of *dispersion*.

The average and other measures of central tendency

Say you were standing with one foot in the oven and one foot in an ice bucket. According to the percentage people, you should be perfectly comfortable.

Bobby Bragan

What was Babe Ruth's batting average? What's the average CEO salary of a Fortune 500 company? What's the average life expectancy for men in the US? Of all summary measurements about a collection, the average is by far the most frequently cited. But to prepare for what's coming later in this chapter, we need to generalize the concept.

The **average** of a collection of numbers (with repeats allowed) is obtained by adding the numbers together and dividing by their total count. The average is also called the **mean** or **expected value** of the collection, and is usually denoted by the Greek letter μ (mu).

For example, if six students take an exam, and one gets a score of 5, three get a score of 6, and two get a score of 8, then the average score is [5 + 6 + 6 + 6 + 8 + 8] / 6 or 6.5. We can rewrite this expression as [5 + (3×6) + (2×8)] / 6. That's not much of savings in length, but with a large number of repeated scores, the savings would be clear.

In general, if the collection contains n_1 occurrences of the value x_1, and n_2 occurrences of the value x_2, and so on up to n_k occurrences of the value x_k, then the mean μ of the collection is:

$$\frac{n_1 x_1 + n_2 x_2 + \cdots + n_k x_k}{N} = \left(\frac{n_1}{N}\right) x_1 + \left(\frac{n_2}{N}\right) x_2 + \cdots + \left(\frac{n_k}{N}\right) x_k$$

where $N = n_1 + n_2 + \cdots + n_k$ is the total number of elements in the collection. If we don't know N or any of the n_j, but do know each fraction $p_j = n_j/N$, then we can still compute the mean μ of the collection as:

$$\mu = p_1 x_1 + p_2 x_2 + \cdots + p_k x_k.$$

Similarly, the above expression is taken to be the mean (average) outcome of a chance experiment whose possible outcome values are $x_1, x_2, \cdots, x_k$ with corresponding probabilities $p_1, p_2, \cdots, p_k$. Similarly, given a probability histogram with bins centered at locations $x_1, x_2, \cdots, x_k$ and corresponding bar probabilities $p_1, p_2, \cdots, p_k$, the above expression is the mean (average) value of the locations.

It can be shown that the mean of a collection of numbers is the value that minimizes the sum of *squared* distances to all the numbers in the collection (and not the value that minimizes the sum of distances to all the numbers in the collection).

Often a chance experiment has one of two possible outcomes: the selected person has the disease or does not; the drug worked on the selected patient or it didn't; the coin toss resulted in a head or a tail. In each case, the two alternatives are typically assigned scores 0 and 1. Suppose that in a population of individuals, a fraction p of them have a score of 1, and the remaining have a score of 0. The mean score of the population is then $(p)(1) + (1 - p)(0) = p$, which is just the *fraction* of the population whose score is 1. Similarly, we can talk about the mean score of a randomly chosen individual from the population: With probability p that score is 1, and with probability $1 - p$ that score is 0. So the mean score is $(p)(1) + (1 - p)(0) = p$.

The average human has one breast and one testicle.

Des McHale

In general, the average (mean) is a measure of **central tendency** of a collection of data, one of several such measures. The term suggests that the number is representative of the data, and that the data is somehow clustered around it. However, viewing the average in this way can sometimes be misleading. For example, a lottery with 100 players might pay a thousand bucks to the holder of the winning ticket and zero to the other 99 ticket holders. The average payout is ten dollars – but that is considerably more than the great majority of players will receive, and so abuses our notion of central tendency.

But one thing for sure about the average: somebody is at least as high and somebody is at least as low. Which makes us smile when Garrison Keillor ends his weekly monologue with: *Well folks, that's the news from Lake Wobegon, where all the women are strong, all the men are good looking, and all the children are above average.*

Even with its shortcomings, the average (mean) is the most quoted measure of central tendency. This is certainly true in medicine: What is the average survival time after a heart transplant? What is the average recovery time from tick fever? What is the average lifetime of this joint replacement? How long is the average wait time for this drug to take effect? When medical data is presented, and a measure of central tendency is called for, it's usually the average that's offered.

Given a collection of numbers arranged from smallest to largest, the **median** is the middle number when the collection is odd, and the halfway-point between the middle numbers when the collection is even. So, the median of the list 0, 2, 2, 5, 6, 7, 18 with seven values is 5. The median of the list 0, 2, 3, 6, 7, 18 with six values is 4.5.

Recalling the example of the previous section in which a lottery with 100 players pays a thousand bucks to the holder of the winning ticket and zero to the other 99 ticket holders, the median winnings is zero. This is certainly more representative of winnings than the mean.

It can be shown that the median of a collection of numbers is the value that minimizes the sum of distances to all the numbers in the collection.

The median is also called the 50th percentile because 50% of the data is below the median and 50% is above. In some applications, we might be interested in other percentiles, maybe the 20th, 40th, 60th, or 80th percentile. The 20th percentile is a mark where 20% of the data is below the mark and 80% is above.

Another measure of central tendency is the **mode**, defined as the number that appears most often in the collection. For example, the collection, 0, 1, 1, 3, 9, 9, 9, 10, has 9 as its mode. But if a collection has two or more modes, it's hard to think of the mode as a measure of central tendency. Also, if the collection consists of the numbers 1 through 9, and two copies of 10, then the mode is 10, and that hardly seems like the center of the list. But in many other situations, the mode does a good job of capturing the idea of center.

When a collection of numbers is widely dispersed or

concentrated at the extremes, a measure of central tendency in itself may not provide a useful characterization or summary of the data. A measure of dispersion in the data can indicate how good is the measure of central tendency. Generally speaking, the greater the dispersion of the data, the less representative is a measure of central tendency.

Variance and standard deviation

The most common measure of dispersion is the **variance**, or its square root, the **standard deviation.** The variance of a collection of numbers (repeats allowed) is defined as the average *squared* distance from the mean to all the numbers in the collection. For example, if the collection consists of the scores 1, 2, 5 and 8, then the mean is 4 and the variance is:

$[(1-4)^2 + (2-4)^2 + (5-4)^2 + (8-4)^2] / 4 = (9 + 4 + 1 + 16) / 4 = 7.5$.

The standard deviation is the square root of this, about 2.74 in this example. The standard deviation of a collection of numbers is usually denoted by the Greek letter σ (sigma), while the variance is denoted σ^2. (The definition of variance involves average *squared* distance rather than average distance because the former has certain nice mathematical properties that the latter does not.)

Suppose we have a collection of N numbers (repeats allowed) with mean μ. Suppose there are n_1 occurrences of the value x_1, and n_2 occurrences of the value x_2, and so on up to n_k occurrences of the value x_k, and we define $p_j = n_j/N$ for each j. Then the variance of the collection is:

$$\sigma^2 = p_1(x_1 - \mu)^2 + p_2(x_2 - \mu)^2 + \cdots + p_k(x_k - \mu)^2$$

And the standard deviation, σ, is the square root of this.

Similarly, the above expression is taken to be the variance of a chance experiment whose possible outcome values are

$x_1, x_2, \cdots, x_k$ with corresponding probabilities $p_1, p_2, \cdots, p_k$. Similarly, given a probability histogram with bins centered at locations $x_1, x_2, \cdots, x_k$, and corresponding bar probabilities $p_1, p_2, \cdots, p_k$, the above expression is the variance of the locations.

The standard deviation of a collection of numbers is expressed in the same units as the numbers themselves. So if the numbers are in meters, then the standard deviation is in meters. If the numbers are in centimeters, the standard deviation is in centimeters. How do you the compare the standard deviations of two different collections when the units are different? You have to convert the units. For example, if one collection has units of pounds and the other has units of kilograms, then we can multiply all the numbers in the second collection by 2.2 pounds/kilo, compute the standard deviation of those numbers, and the result will be in pounds. Or more simply, we could just multiply the standard deviation of the second collection by 2.2 pounds/kilo to get the equivalent standard deviation in pounds.

Suppose that in a population of individuals, a fraction p of them have a score of 1, and the remaining have a score of 0. We saw previously that the mean score is then p. What is the variance of the scores? For the fraction p who have a score of 1, the squared distance to the mean is $(1-p)^2$. For the fraction $1-p$ who have a score of 0, the squared distance to the mean is $(0-p)^2 = p^2$. So, the variance of the population is $(1-p)p^2 + p(1-p)^2$, which simplifies to $p(1-p)$. Similarly, we can talk about the variance of the score of a randomly chosen individual from the population: Again the variance of the score is $p(1-p)$. This value is always between 0 and 0.25, and so the standard deviation is always between 0 and 0.5.

Given a population of scores that are between 0 and 1, the variance of the population is again between 0 and 0.25.

Suppose you learn that a hip replacement has an average lifetime (the duration over which no surgical revision is required) of 15 years. Should you be satisfied with that as a characterization of how well hip replacement surgery performs? You should not. You should ask about the standard deviation. You might inquire about the median. Even better, a probability histogram for hip replacement lifetime will tell you many things you should know.

Mean and variance for distribution curves

We've seen how to compute the mean and variance for probability histograms. Using the calculus, we can also compute mean and variance for probability distribution curves. (The general idea is to approximate the region under the curve by a probability histogram that has a gazillion bars, and then compute the mean and variance of that histogram.)

Among probability distributions encountered in practice, none occurs more often than the bell-shaped distribution – also known as the **Normal** distribution. See Figure 9-1. (An example of this distribution was shown earlier in Figure 7-1.) The shape of a Normal distribution is fully determined by μ and σ, its mean and

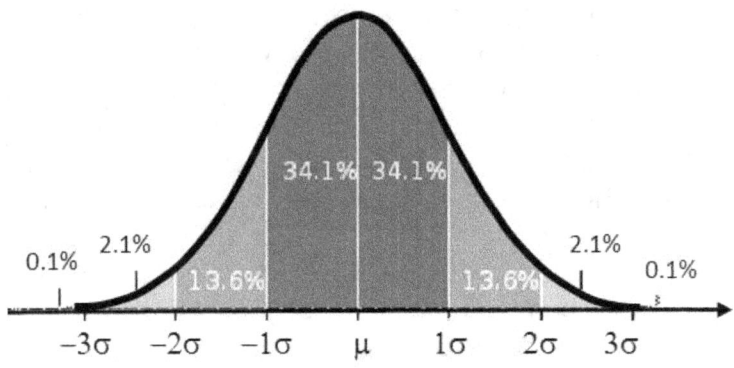

Figure 9-1 *A Normal distribution with mean μ and standard deviation σ, showing the amount of area (probability) captured within 1, 2, and 3 standard deviations of the mean.*

standard deviation, and so is often denoted by the symbol $N(\mu, \sigma)$. In particular, the Normal distribution with mean $\mu = 0$ and standard deviation $\sigma = 1$ is called the **Standard Normal** distribution, denoted $N(0, 1)$. Regarding the Normal distribution $N(\mu, \sigma)$, the interval $[\mu - \sigma, \mu + \sigma]$ always captures 68.2% of the area; the interval $[\mu - 2\sigma, \mu + 2\sigma]$ always captures 95.4% of the area; and the interval $[\mu - 3\sigma, \mu + 3\sigma]$ always captures 99.6% of the area.

The probabilities, 68.2%, 95.4%, and 99.6%, captured by the intervals above are not necessarily the probabilities captured by these same intervals when applied to other distributions. For example, consider a probability distribution that has three "narrow spikes" of probability: a spike with 49% probability at location -1 on the horizontal axis, a spike with 49% probability at location $+1$, and a third spike with 2% probability at location 0. The mean μ of this distribution is 0 and the standard deviation σ is a little less than 1. This distribution has only 2% of its probability in the interval $[\mu - \sigma, \mu + \sigma]$.

Mean and variance in higher dimensions

So far we have been considering one-dimensional data, involving one type of measurement, such as a set of IQ's, or a set of body weights, or a set of longevities. But often the data that we need to analyze is more complicated, involving pairs or triples of measurements simultaneously. For example, we may want to see how age and resting pulse rate are jointly distributed in a population, or how HDL, LDL, and triglyceride readings are jointly distributed in a population. When considering pairs of measurements, we're looking at data points in two-dimensional space. When considering triples of measurements, we're looking at data points in three-dimensional space. So we need to extend the notions of mean and variance to deal with multi-dimensional data.

The mean of a two-dimensional data set – that is to say, the mean of a set of pairs (x, y) – is taken to be (μ_x, μ_y), where μ_x is the mean of the x measurements, and μ_y is the mean of the y measurements. The mean of a three-dimensional data set (or higher-dimensional data set) is similarly defined.

The notion of variance extends to two and higher dimensions, but not as directly as the mean. In two and higher dimensions, the analog of variance is a table of numbers called the *covariance matrix*. In one dimension, the variance σ^2 leads to an interval $[\mu - \sigma, \mu + \sigma]$ about the mean. In two dimensions, the covariance matrix leads to an *ellipse* about the mean. In higher dimensions, the covariance matrix leads to an *ellipsoid* about the mean.

The Binomial distribution

Besides the Normal distribution, another distribution that commonly occurs in practice is the *Binomial*. It plays an important role in sampling.

Suppose an urn contains N marbles, a fraction p of them white and the remaining black. Suppose that n marbles are selected from the urn at random. (They may be selected all at once or in succession *without replacement*.) What is the probability that k marbles in the sample are white? Equivalently, what proportion of samples with n marbles have k of them white? An exact formula is known, but it's a bit unwieldy, so we'll content ourselves with a close approximation. If the number N of marbles in the urn is much larger than the sample size n (and p is not "too close" to 0 or 1), then the probability that k marbles in the sample are white turns out to be well-approximated by the formula

$$B(n,p,k) = \langle n,k \rangle p^k (1-p)^{n-k}.$$

Here the symbol $\langle n, k \rangle$, read "n choose k", denotes the number of k-element subsets that can be drawn from an n-element set. (This symbol was first mentioned in Example 4 of Chapter 7.) Notice that the above formula does not depend on the parameter N (the number of marbles in the urn), but only on the parameters n, p, and k.

Though $B(n, p, k)$ is an approximate formula for our question at hand, it is an *exact* formula for two related experiments: (1) $B(n, p, k)$ is the exact probability that k marbles are white among a sample of n marbles drawn from the urn at random *with replacement* (i.e., drawn in succession with each marble returned to the urn before the next one is drawn); (2) $B(n, p, k)$ is the *exact* probability that k heads occur in n tosses of a biased coin, where p is the probability that a single toss of the coin comes up heads.

Why is $B(n, p, k)$ an exact formula for these latter two experiments? Referring to the marble selection experiment with replacement: There are $\langle n, k \rangle$ ways of picking k positions for the white marbles in a sequence of n total marbles and each such configuration occurs with the probability $p^k(1-p)^{n-k}$. A similar explanation holds for the coin tossing experiment.

If we fix the parameters n and p, and let k vary as $0, 1, 2,\ldots, n$, then the **Binomial** distribution, denoted $B(n, p)$, associates the value $B(n, p, k)$ with each value of k. This distribution is conveniently depicted as a histogram with $n + 1$ bars centered at locations $0, 1, 2,\ldots, n$ on the horizontal axis, where the area of bar k is $B(n, p, k)$ for each k, and the width of each bar is 1.

If you Google, "SticiGui Binomial Probability Histogram", you can interact with a Binomial histogram widget and see what the histogram looks like for different values of n and p.

A related distribution, what we'll call the **fractional Binomial** distribution, denoted $FB(n, p)$, associates the value $B(n, p, k)$ with each *fraction* k/n of white marbles in the sample. It has a histogram just like that of the Binomial $B(n, p)$, the same bar areas as before, but now the bars are centered at locations, $0, 1/n, 2/n,\ldots, (n-1)/n, 1$ on the horizontal axis, and the width of each bar is taken to be $1/n$. (We'll see pictures in the next section.)

It can be shown that the fractional Binomial $FB(n, p)$ histogram has mean p and variance $p(1-p)/n$. For fixed sample size n, this variance is greatest when $p = 0.5$ and decreases to 0 as p tends toward 0 or 1. No matter what p is, we see that this variance (which reflects the "width" of the histogram) goes to zero as the sample size n increases.

Suppose we're presented with a large 0-1 population (i.e., a large population of 0's and 1's) whose mean is p. If a sample of size n is drawn from this population, and the number of 1's in that sample is k, then the mean of the sample is k/n. Consider the histogram that indicates, for each value k/n (with k varying 0, 1, 2,..., n), the proportion of samples of size n whose mean is k/n. Then this **histogram of sample means** is well-approximated by the fractional Binomial histogram $FB(n, p)$, being analogous to the situation with marbles above. So when we speak of the histogram of sample means, we're essentially speaking of the fractional Binomial histogram $FB(n, p)$.

Probability concentration about the mean

What does the fractional Binomial histogram $FB(n, p)$ look like for different values of p and sample size n? Figure 9-2 shows three fractional Binomials, each with $p = 0.5$ and different values for n. Each is a probability histogram, and so has area one.

Figure 9-2 suggests that as n increases, the fractional Binomial histogram $FB(n, p = 0.5)$ concentrates more and more of its area (probability) into any fixed *positive-length* interval $[0.5 - a, 0.5 + a]$ about the histogram mean $p = 0.5$, and that this area is going to 1. In fact, this **concentration of probability about the mean** can be proven mathematically. (It's a consequence of the fact that the variance of the fractional Binomial goes to 0 as n increases.) It follows that for any value c less than 1, there is a smallest value for n such that the amount of histogram area within the fixed interval $[0.5 - a, 0.5 + a]$ is at least c. (Note: It can be shown that as n increases, the probability associated with the centermost histogram bar goes to 0. That's why the interval mentioned above has to be of positive length.)

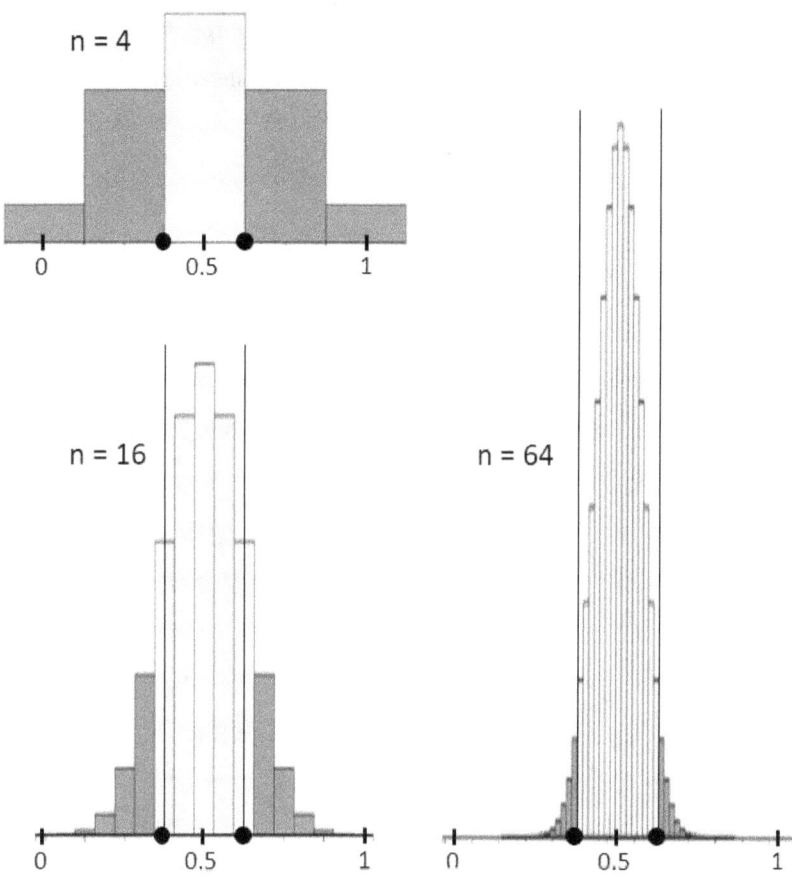

Figure 9-2 *The fractional Binomial histogram FB(n, p = 0.5) for different values of n. Here the black dots delimit the fixed interval [0.5 − a, 0.5 + a] where a = 0.125.*

Since concentration of probability holds for the fractional Binomial $FB(n, p = 0.5)$, it holds for the histogram of sample means (for samples of size n) associated with a large 0-1 population whose population mean is 0.5. This implies that for any value c less than 1, there is a smallest sample size n such that the proportion of samples of size n with mean inside the interval $[0.5 - a, 0.5 + a]$ is at least c. For this sample size n, the probability that a randomly chosen sample has its mean within the interval $[0.5 - a, 0.5 + a]$ is at least c.

Now consider Figure 9-3, which shows three fractional Binomials $FB(n, p)$, each with $p = 0.75$ and different values for n. Once again, we see that the histogram $FB(n, p = 0.75)$ displays concentration of probability about its mean, $p = 0.75$, as n increases. (Note: $FB(n, p = 0.75)$ is *asymmetric* for all n, but becomes more symmetric as n increases.)

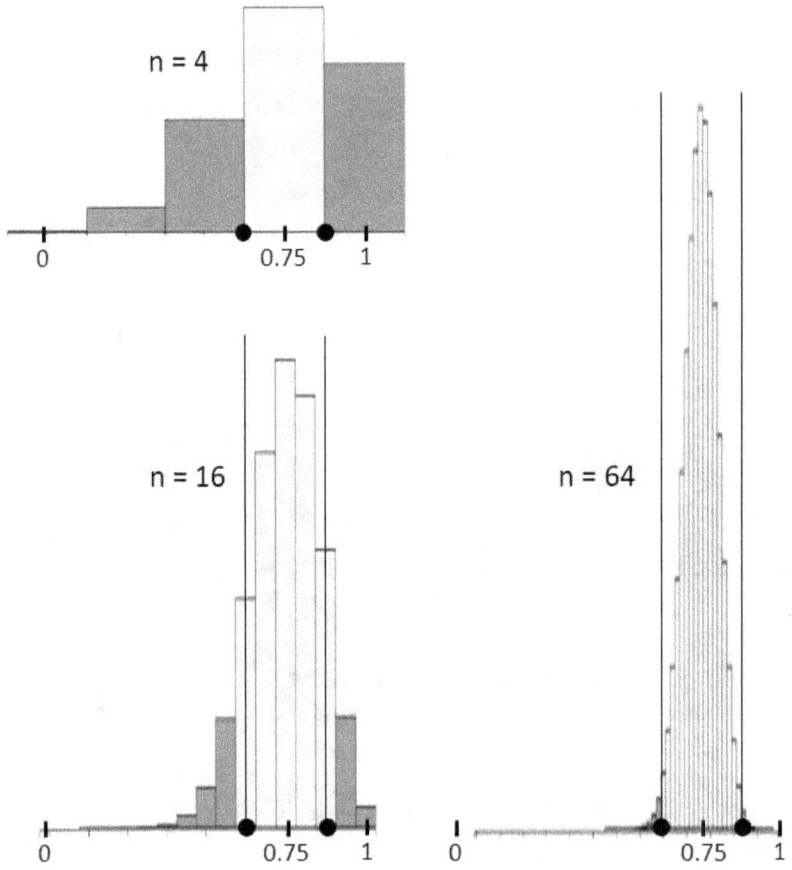

Figure 9-3 *The fractional Binomial histogram FB(n, p = 0.75) for different values of n. Here the black dots delimit the fixed interval [0.75 − a, 0.75 + a] where a = 0.125.*

In fact, for any value of p strictly between 0 and 1, it can be shown that the fractional Binomial $FB(n, p)$ demonstrates concentration of probability about its mean p as n increases. (While for $p = 0$ or $p = 1$, concentration of probability is immediate.) This concentration justifies the statement: The greater the sample size, the greater the proportion of samples that are representative of the population, and hence the more likely that a randomly chosen sample is representative of the population. Given the values of a, c, and p, a computer can easily calculate the smallest value of n such that the area of the fractional Binomial $FB(n, p)$ contained within the interval $[p - a, p + a]$ is at least c.

(*For the advanced reader*: An approximation to this smallest value of n is provided by a formula that derives from the *Central Limit Theorem* (CLT). This theorem shows that for any given p greater than 0 and less than 1, the fractional Binomial $FB(n, p)$ is better and better approximated by a Normal distribution as n increases. Without going into details, the *CLT sample size formula* (when p is known) is the following:

$$n = \frac{(x(c))^2 p(1-p)}{a^2}$$

Here $x(c)$ is the number such that the interval $[-x(c), +x(c)]$ captures area c under the Standard Normal distribution. An online Normal distribution calculator can compute $x(c)$ for any value of c less than 1. For example, if $c = 0.95$, then $x(c) = 1.96$.

The formula above is only an *approximation*. It's considered a good approximation when p is in a certain "safe zone" (depending on a and c) that is not "too close" to 0 or 1. Otherwise it's a poor approximation. If $a = 0.05$, $c = 0.95$, and $p = 0.5$, then p happens to be in the safe zone, and $n = 384$ turns out to be the approximate smallest sample size. If instead, $p = 0.75$, then p is also in the safe zone, and $n = 288$ is the approximate smallest sample size.)

Concentration of probability about the mean generalizes to populations other than 0-1 populations. Suppose we're dealing with any large population of measurements (e.g., body weight) with population mean µ. If we were to form the "distribution of sample means" from all samples of size n, we would again see a concentration of probability about the mean µ as n increases. In this general context, the concentration phenomenon is usually referred to as the *Law of Large Numbers*.

Concentration of probability about the mean generalizes to higher dimensions: Suppose we're dealing with a large population of measurement pairs (x, y), whose mean is $(µ_x, µ_y)$. If we were to form the "distribution of sample means" from all samples of size n, we would see a concentration of probability about the mean $(µ_x, µ_y)$ as n increases.

Sample size to estimate a population mean

Suppose we're presented with a large 0-1 population and we want to estimate the *unknown* population mean p by computing the mean of a randomly chosen sample. Of course, we want the sample to be as small as possible. On the other hand, the sample has to be large enough so that the estimate satisfies certain "accuracy" and "confidence" requirements. What is meant by these terms?

We say that a sample estimate of the population mean p of a 0-1 population is within 5% **absolute accuracy** if the estimate lies within the interval $[p - 0.05, p + 0.05]$. We say that a sample estimate for p is within 5% **relative accuracy** if the estimate lies within the interval $[p - (0.05)p, p + (0.05)p]$. Absolute accuracy involves an interval whose length does not depend on p, while relative accuracy involves an interval whose length does depend on p and goes to zero as p goes to zero. From here on, we'll use the term **accuracy** to mean absolute accuracy.

What is meant by the term "confidence"? We say, for example, that a sample size n provides an estimate for p that is within 3% accuracy at 95% **confidence** if among all samples of size n, the proportion of them that have sample mean in the interval $[p - 0.03, p + 0.03]$ is at least 95%. Or said another way: the probability that a random sample of size n has sample mean in the interval $[p - 0.03, p + 0.03]$ is at least 95%.

In general, for any specified accuracy a greater than 0 and confidence c less than 1, we say that a sample size n is **(a, c)-good** for estimating the population mean p if among all samples of size n, the proportion of them having mean within the interval $[p - a, p + a]$ is at least c. Equivalently, we say that the sample size n is (a, c)-good for estimating p if the probability that a random sample of size n has mean within the interval $[p - a, p + a]$ is at least c. A fixed sample size n is (a, c)-good for various combinations of a and c, where the larger the a, the larger the c, i.e., the lower the accuracy the higher the confidence.

Suppose we have a large 0-1 population with unknown mean p. Fix a sample size n. Pick an accuracy a such that at least 95% of samples of size n have their sample mean within accuracy a of the population mean. Then for those same 95% of samples, the population mean is within accuracy a of the sample mean. Equivalently, for this sample size n and accuracy a, if we grab a random sample of size n and denote its mean by $\hat{p}$ (read "p hat"), then there is a 95% chance that the population mean p lies in the interval $[\hat{p} - a, \hat{p} + a]$. This interval about the sample mean $\hat{p}$ is called a 95% **confidence interval** for estimating the population mean. Similarly, we can speak of a 70% confidence interval, an 80% confidence interval, an 85% confidence interval, and so on.

Confidence intervals are crucial for helping us judge the reliability of statistical (i.e., sample-based) estimates. If someone hands you an estimate of a population mean without handing you a defensible confidence interval, then you shouldn't give the estimate much credence.

Given accuracy a greater than 0 and confidence c less than 1, and a large 0-1 population with unknown mean p, what is the smallest sample size n that is (a, c)-good for estimating p? **Equivalently:** Given accuracy a and confidence c, what is the smallest sample size n such that the area of the fractional Binomial

$FB(n, p)$ within the interval $[p - a, p + a]$ is at least c, *no matter what* value of p is being considered? First of all, does such a sample size even exist? The answer is yes. (It's a consequence of the fact that the biggest variance a fractional Binomial can have is $0.25/n$, which occurs when $p = 0.5$, and this variance goes to 0 as n increases.) In what follows, we're going to describe an "exact method" for getting this smallest sample size.

Here's the strategy: Consider, say, a thousand equally-spaced candidate values of p between 0 and 1. For each candidate p, find the smallest sample size n such that the area of the fractional Binomial $FB(n, p)$ histogram within the interval $[p - a, p + a]$ is at least c. Among all these pairs (p, n), identify the one that has the maximum value of n. This is the sample size n we seek. This algorithm can be run by computer.

(*For the advanced reader*: For fixed accuracy a and confidence c, the smallest sample size n that is (a, c)-good for estimating the unknown mean of a large 0-1 population is approximated by the CLT sample size formula of the previous section upon plugging in the value of p that makes the formula attain its maximum value. That occurs when setting p equal to 0.5. So, the smallest sample size n that is (a, c)-good for estimating the unknown mean of a large 0-1 population is *approximately* given by the *CLT sample size formula*:

$$n = \frac{(x(c))^2 (0.25)}{a^2}$$

This approximation is considered good as long as the unknown population mean p we're trying to estimate is in the "safe zone" (depending on a and c) mentioned in the previous section. Using the above formula, if $a = 5\%$ and $c = 95\%$, then $n = 384$ is the approximate smallest sample size. If $a = 3\%$ and $c = 95\%$, then $n = 1067$ is the approximate smallest sample size. The formula can also be viewed as an approximate relationship between sample size and confidence intervals – given sample size n, it tells us what combinations of a and c render the sample size (a, c)-good for estimating the population mean.

The authors do not know if the CLT sample size formula gives the same result as the exact method, the latter providing valid answers without any constraints on p.)

In some applications, the goal is to obtain an (a, c)-good estimate of the unknown mean p of a large 0-1 population, where a is intended to be *relative* accuracy instead of absolute accuracy. Such a sample size n exists only when p is presumed to be within an interval $[b, 1]$, where b is bigger than zero. In this case, finding the exact smallest sample size n that is (a, c)-good for estimating p can be accomplished using a small modification of the exact method mentioned earlier.

If a sample size n is (a, c)-good for estimating the unknown mean p of a large 0-1 population, then the same sample size is (a, c)-good for estimating the unknown mean μ of any large population of measurements that are *between* 0 and 1. The authors admit they know only an intuitive explanation for this statement rather than a mathematical proof. (The intuition follows from this: Among all populations of N measurements in the interval $[0, 1]$ with mean μ, it can be shown that the distribution of sample means has the largest standard deviation when the population consists only of 0's and 1's.)

What about measurements outside the interval $[0, 1]$? Suppose we're presented with a large population of measurements in the range $[L, R]$ that has unknown mean μ. If m is a measurement in the interval $[L, R]$, then $m^* = (m - L)/(R - L)$ transforms that measurement to a number within the interval $[0, 1]$. It follows that if the sample size n is (a, c)-good for estimating the population mean of the transformed measurements, it is (a^*, c)-good for estimating the mean of the original measurements, where $a^* = a \times (R - L)$.

Confidence interval explained in a nutshell

Suppose we wish to understand the success rate of a particular treatment for a particular kind of patient. Say we go to a nationwide database of electronic medical records and discover that there are 100 patients of this kind in the database who have received the treatment. We then run a statistical analysis on this sample and the final report tells us that a fraction 0.7 (i.e., 70%) of the member patients had success with the treatment, and that the predicted success rate in general for this kind of patient is 0.7 with 95% confidence interval [0.7 − 0.1, 0.7 + 0.1]. A friend looking over our shoulder asks, "What is meant by this confidence interval?"

It can be explained briefly as follows: To our knowledge, the presence of the 100 patients in the database did not depend on treatment outcome − the patients were not filtered in any way to decide inclusion in the database. So the 100 patients can be reasonably viewed as an unbiased sample from among the population of all patients (of the particular kind) who either did receive or will receive the treatment. It's as if, among all possible samples of size 100, we picked one of these samples at random. The goal of the analysis is to estimate the population success rate from the sample success rate. Rock-solid, incontrovertible mathematics guarantees that 95% of samples of size 100 have their sample success rate within 0.1 of the population success rate. So the odds that the sample in the database is one of these "representative" samples is 95%.

If there were more than 100 patients (of the particular kind) in the database, and we picked 100 from them arbitrarily, and if 70% of those had success with the treatment, then we would still have the same 95% confidence interval, [0.7 − 0.1, 0.7 + 0.1], justified by the same explanation.

Confidence interval from sample size and mean

Suppose we're presented with a large 0-1 population and we want to estimate the unknown population mean p. Suppose the sample size n and desired confidence level c have been dictated to us. Note, the sample size n could be quite small, as occurs, for example, when only few patients are available for a study, or only limited funding is available to for the study. Suppose we draw an unbiased (random) sample of size n from the population and observe its mean, which we denote as $\hat{p}$. What is the tightest accuracy a such that this sample mean is (a, c)-good for estimating the population mean?

A solution can be obtained using the exact method. Consider a bunch of candidate values for p between 0 and 1. For each candidate, determine the smallest value of a such that the area of the fractional Binomial $FB(n, p)$ within the interval $[p - a, p + a]$ is at least c. Among the pairs (p, a) such that the aforementioned interval contains $\hat{p}$, identify the one with largest value of a. This is the accuracy a that we seek, making $[\hat{p} - a, \hat{p} + a]$ into a c confidence interval about the observed sample mean.

It can be argued that this value of a works even for a population of measurements between 0 and 1. In this latter scenario, additional math explores the use of the observed sample standard deviation to tighten the confidence interval further.

Statistical hypothesis testing

Instead of trying to estimate the unknown mean p of a large 0-1 population, we may already have an hypothesis regarding the value of p, and may want to see if there is compelling statistical evidence to reject the hypothesis. Absent such evidence, we should consider the hypothesis to be *potentially* true.

Suppose we hypothesize that a certain coin is fair, i.e., that the probability of tossing heads with this coin is 0.5. The only way to test this hypothesis is to toss the coin some number of times and see what ratio of heads to total tosses we get. However, with a large number of tosses, it's unlikely that precisely half the tosses will be heads, even if the coin is fair. In fact, assuming an even number n of tosses, the probability that exactly half the tosses will come up heads goes to zero as n increases! So what good are repeated tosses of the coin in testing the hypothesis?

Returning to Figure 9-2 we see that for a fair coin, the ratio of heads to total tosses is more likely to be close to 0.5 the more times n that we toss the coin. In fact, the probability that the ratio is between, say, 0.45 and 0.55 goes to 1 as n increases.

It can be shown that when n is roughly 384, this probability is at least 95%. So, if after 384 tosses you observe the ratio to be outside the interval [0.45, 0.55], you have good grounds to reject the fair-coin hypothesis – in fact, you can be 95% confident in the correctness of that conclusion. That's because there is only a 5% probability by chance alone that a fair coin tossed 384 times would yield an observed ratio outside the interval [0.45, 0.55].

On the other hand, if after 384 tosses you observe the ratio to be within the interval [0.45, 0.55], you *cannot* take that as proof that the coin is fair. In fact, no matter how many times the coin is tossed, and no matter what the outcome, you can never be absolutely certain that the coin is fair. But, by sampling, you might be able to say with great confidence (though short of 100%) that if the coin is biased, it's biased by at most a "small" amount, "small" being other than 0 but of your choosing.

Suppose we hypothesize that the prevalence of a particular harm among those taking a certain drug is no more than one in a thousand, that is to say, no more than 0.001. Let's see how statistics can be used to test the validity of this hypothesis.

Suppose that within the population of those taking the drug, a score of 1 is associated with anyone who incurs the harm, and a score of 0 is associated with anyone who does not. The population mean is then the prevalence of the harm in the population. Set accuracy a to be, say, 0.0005, and set confidence

c to be, say, 95%. Pretend for the moment that the population mean is exactly the hypothesized maximum 0.001. Determine the smallest sample size n such that the area of the fractional Binomial $FB(n, p = 0.001)$ to the left of $0.001 + 0.0005$ (i.e., 0.0015) is at least 95%. See Figure 9-4. For this sample size, if the population mean were between 0 and 0.001, then with probability at least 95%, the sample mean would be less than 0.0015. It follows that if you select a random sample of size n and you observe the sample mean to be greater than 0.0015, then you can reject the hypothesis at the 95% confidence level. (If the hypothesis were true, then you must have picked a rare sample, one of the "bad" 5% of samples – which is unlikely. That said, the decision to reject the hypothesis based on this bad sample is wrong 5% of the time in a well-defined sense.) Otherwise, you should view the hypothesis as being potentially true.

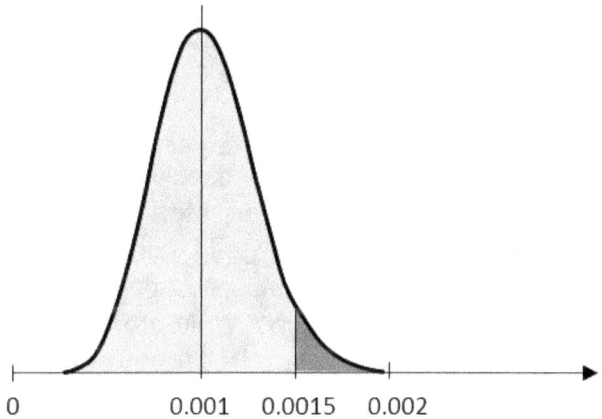

Figure 9-4 *The fractional Binomial histogram FB(n, p = 0.001) with sample size n chosen so that the area to the left of 0.0015 is 0.95.*

Conversely, suppose we hypothesize that a new drug will be at least 10% effective for people with a certain disease. The approach of this section gives us a way of quantifying the plausibility of that hypothesis.

Estimating things besides a population mean

In some applications, it's not the population mean that we want to estimate, but the population median or standard deviation. Of course, we want the estimate to satisfy certain accuracy and confidence requirements. Fortunately, there's mathematics similar to what we've seen that tells us the requisite sample sizes.

In other applications, we want to estimate a histogram or bar chart related to the population. If it's a histogram we're after, then we need a sample size that allows us to simultaneously estimate, at desired confidence, the areas of all bars to within desired accuracy. A histogram should always be accompanied by a "confidence envelope" if it is being used to make predictions about a larger population. If it's a bar chart we're after, then we need a sample size (per bin) that allows us to simultaneously estimate, at desired confidence, the heights of all bars to within requisite accuracy. Again, there's mathematics to tell us the requisite sample size. A bar chart should always be accompanied by a "confidence envelope" if it is being used to make predictions about a larger population.

Suppose a medical test has been developed that indicates whether or not a patient has a certain disease. We'd like to know the quality of this test. If there is a gold standard to compare against, we can ask the following questions: What is the sensitivity and specificity of the test? What are its positive and negative prediction values? What are its false positive and false negative rates? We'd like to know each of these to within requisite accuracy and confidence. Again, there's mathematics to tell us the requisite sample sizes.

Watson guarding the old guard

In 2011, with much hoopla and fanfare, IBM's Watson became the first machine to win *Jeopardy!*, trouncing its human competitors in real-time. It was considered a milestone in machine intelligence and natural language processing (NLP). For those not familiar with *Jeopardy!*, it is a popular television gameshow that first aired in 1964. Contestants are shown general knowledge clues in the form of answers, and they have to respond to these clues in the form of questions. (In *Jeopardy!*, the answer begs the question.) The correct response may require an understanding of metaphor, idiom, sarcasm, and other subtleties that enliven natural language.

Flush with their *Jeopardy!* success, IBM turned to monetizing Watson in the realms of business, law, finance, and medicine. In each domain, Watson is being tailored to answer questions of a diverse and complex nature, and the information it has to work from is typically expressed in natural language.

For applications in clinical medicine, Watson is being primed for the role of expert advisor, helping the doctor identify best treatment options for the individual patient. A particular focus area is cancer. For example, IBM and Memorial Sloan Kettering (MSK) Cancer Center are partnering in the development of Watson for Oncology. Up to 2017, MD Anderson Cancer Center was leveraging Watson in its development of the Oncology Expert Advisor. In this paradigm, Watson ingests the patient's EMR, extracts the relevant details, and then probes for answers about treatment in a vast archive of information that includes medical journals, textbooks, clinical rationales, consensus guidelines, news reports, clinical trials, and other patients' medical records. According to IBM, Watson for Oncology draws from a corpus of over 290 medical journals, 200 textbooks, and 12 million pages of text. Most of these sources are a mixture of structured and unstructured data. The patient's EMR is of such nature: the structured part consists of data fields with coded answers; the unstructured part consists of doctor's notes, medical images, ECG readings, and the like.

In a 2104 YouTube video titled, "IBM Watson: How it Works", IBM explains the Watson technical approach to clinical medicine (italics are quotes from the video):

To begin, Watson is provided a "corpus of knowledge"

curated by human experts. These experts *cull through the information, discarding anything that is out-of-date, poorly-regarded, or immaterial to the problem domain.*

After ingesting the corpus, human experts train Watson on *how to interpret the information. Experts upload training data into Watson in the form of question-answer pairs. Interactions between users and Watson are periodically reviewed by experts and fed back into the system to help Watson better interpret information. Likewise as new information is published, Watson is updated so that it is constantly adapting to shifts in knowledge.*

Watson is now ready to respond to questions about highly complex situations and quickly provide a range of potential responses and recommendations that are backed by evidence. It is also prepared to identify new insights or patterns locked away in information.

For each recommendation, Watson scores it using various contextual and linguistic algorithms. It then combines these scores into a single score, between zero and one, that IBM refers to as the "confidence" of the recommendation. If the confidence is below a threshold, the recommendation is discarded. The remaining recommendations are ranked by the confidence and presented to the doctor, along with links to supporting evidence. Doctors can now (quote) *judge the clinical relevance of the data and make their own treatment decisions.*

Two major themes stand out in IBM's pitch of Watson to the medical profession: deference to the human expert and heavy reliance on published content. Statistical analysis applied directly to historical patient outcome data in EMR's is not advertised as being the key driver in Watson's recommendations.

The approach begs a number of questions:

Who curates the curators? Who are the experts? Certainly the term "expert" doesn't have much meaning when considered independent of outcome data. Many so-called experts have gotten it wrong so often that it belies the term. Many so-called experts have gotten it wrong for money and position, pushing unnecessary surgeries and procedures, or pimping for Big Pharma.

Many experts recommended the PSA test as a routine screening tool for prostate cancer, and performed lots of prostate surgeries. Now it's recognized that the PSA test led to massive rates of over-treatment, and it is no longer advised for most men. Many experts recommended hormone replacement therapy to treat the symptoms of menopause. Now we know this therapy leads to serious health risks, and is no longer advised for most women. Many experts recommended mastectomy or lumpectomy for stage 0 breast cancer. But, recent evidence suggests that this is not the best way to proceed – that a more conservative approach is better advised. Many experts recommend stent insertion and angioplasty for unblocking coronary arties, even though there is ample evidence that these do little to reduce mortality.

How does Watson deal with experts who disagree? How are different expert opinions weighted? How is the literature weighted – does it bury the new beneath the mass of the old? When, and under what rules, are old results and old-guard experts phased out in favor of newer results and newer experts?

How much faith should doctor and patient put in the mysterious "confidence" measure that Watson assigns to a recommendation? This measure comes from a black box with no guarantee of reliability or relevance. It is not a statistical characterization of the performance of the treatment. When Watson assigns 75% confidence to a treatment, it doesn't mean that 75% of historical patients had success with this treatment, or anything like that. The utility of Watson's confidence measure is not established.

Does Memorial-Sloan-Kettering's Watson for Oncology give the same answers as MD Anderson's Oncology Expert Advisor? After all, they use different experts. Do these systems give the same answers as other clinical decision support systems – say, for example, the one from QPID Health or DeepMind Health? If they don't give the same answers, how do we decide which system is the more credible?

Back to the Future:

Before entering this section, we were introduced to the basic concepts and methodology of *rigorous statistics*. Recapping: The main ideas were to gather unbiased samples, compute summary information (e.g., mean, histogram) on those samples, and report the information with confidence intervals. Application of rigorous statistics to historical patient data enables objective, quantitative comparisons among treatment options. This is the best way to help patients determine which options are most likely to meet their goals.

In contrast to systems like Watson, the paradigm of rigorous statistics does not rely on subjective expert opinion. Instead, it lets historical patient outcomes do all the talking. The paradigm is not mysterious. It's not a black-box whose ruminations are beyond scrutiny and comprehension, assigning peculiar "confidence" measures to treatment recommendations. Instead, the paradigm delivers an objective quantification of past treatment performance and provides a transparent, well-understood characterization of how well past performance predicts future performance. Moreover, the paradigm lays bare which treatments are superior and which are inferior at the earliest possible time, well before the journal publications or news reports come out.

But the rigorous statistical paradigm requires a change in mindset, and an understanding of basic statistical concepts. The paradigm points to objective truths in patient outcome data. For doctors, sometimes these may be inconvenient truths. But truths in many realms are often inconvenient. Medical decisions should not be based on stale and unsupportable beliefs, habit, hearsay, intuition, heuristics, or on feeding the bottom line. They should be driven by consideration for what's best for the patient in accord with the patient's goals.

Why is the medical profession more receptive to Watson than real-time rigorous statistical analysis? Watson makes few if any demands on the doctor's training, practice style, or time. It does not require a change in the doctor's mindset or view of what constitutes evidence-based medicine. Most physicians have had little training in statistics, and Watson doesn't challenge the physician to understand basic statistical concepts. Watson gathers the latest published information on behalf of the busy doctor, and ultimately defers to the doctor on its clinical relevance. Watson does not challenge the physician's authority or expertise; nor is it seen as vying for the doctor's job.

Postscript:

MD Anderson Cancer Center and IBM launched the joint venture to develop the Watson-based Oncology Expert Advisor in 2013. By early 2017, MD Anderson cancelled the effort because it could not be demonstrated (using rigorous statistics) that the technology improved patient outcomes compared to the usual way doctors arrive at cancer treatment decisions. It appears that IBM greatly over-hyped the Watson technology, while journalists, not doing due diligence in demanding evidential support, were taken for a ride. (See the online article, "MD Anderson Cancer Center's IBM Watson Project Fails, and So Did Journalism Related to It", *Health News Review*, Feb. 23, 2017. See also the online article, "Why Everyone Is Hating on IBM Watson – Including the People Who Helped Make It", *Gizmodo*, Aug. 10, 2017.)

Combining data

A **meta-analysis** (or **meta-study**) is an analysis of analyses – multiple studies are combined with the goal of obtaining more reliable conclusions about an overall population. The pursuit has become increasingly popular thanks to the large number of existing studies and their easy access on the Internet. Although meta-analysis has generated mountains of research papers, the methodology has its pitfalls, and caution is advised in accepting any of its conclusions.

Here's a simple experiment that could form the basis of a meta-study. Suppose we want to determine if an old beat-up coin is fair. We have a friend Joe who flips the coin 20 times, and with each toss, he records whether it lands heads or tails. Suppose the coin comes up heads 15 times. Then Joe goes out for a few beers, comes back, tosses the coin 80 more times, and gets 40 heads among these new tosses. If we are forced to guess the bias of the coin, should we conclude that the probability of heads is ¾ (going with the first set of tosses) or ½ (going with the second set of tosses)?

Or should we combine (pool) the two sessions together, giving 55 heads out of 100 tosses and estimate the bias as 11/20? After all, it's safe to assume that the laws of physics didn't change during Joe's beer-break nor did the properties of the coin. But is it safe to assume that Joe didn't change, that the beer didn't affect his coin-tossing thumb?

The question is not as silly as it might sound. Various laboratory experiments show that people tend to introduce bias in their tosses of a fair coin. Some people toss the coin in such a way that the majority of tosses land with the same face up as when the coin was placed on the thumb; others show the reverse. So, it might be argued that pooling the results of Joe's two sessions isn't meaningful; that they should be kept separate.

Now if Joe went for bottled water instead of beer, maybe the two sessions can be pooled with more confidence. In that case, the estimated bias of the coin would be (15 + 40) / (20 + 80) which equals 55/100, which also equals [(20/100) × (15/20)] + [(80/100) × (40/80)]. In other words, pooling the two sessions gives the same answer as a certain weighted sum of the session means. (The session means are 15/20 and 40/80, and the corresponding weights, 20/100 and 80/100, are the session sizes over the pool size.)

Let's look at another experiment that could form the basis of a meta-study. Suppose we have two disjoint random samples, S_A and S_B, from a large population of measurements. Then each sample mean is an estimate of the population mean with its own confidence interval. It's certainly reasonable to consider pooling the two samples together. This gives a larger random sample with smaller (tighter) confidence interval than either of the original samples. As with the coin experiment above, the estimate of population mean from the pooled sample equals a weighted sum of the original sample means, where the corresponding weights are the sample sizes over the pool size.

Here's yet another example that could form the basis of a meta-study. Suppose a large population of measurements consists of two disjoint subpopulations, A and B. Let S_A denote a random sample from A, and S_B denote a random sample from B. Suppose we want to use these samples to estimate the overall population mean. Is that possible, and can we assign a justified confidence interval? Yes, if we know the fraction f_A of the population that resides in A (and hence the fraction f_B of the population that resides in B). To estimate the overall population mean, compute the product f_A times the sample mean of S_A, and add to it the product f_B times the sample mean of S_B. It can be shown that this estimate comes with a rigorous, quantifiable confidence interval. But if f_A and f_B are not known, then all bets are off – we are not aware of a rigorous way to combine the results of the two samples to get an estimate of the population mean whose reliability can be quantified.

Many meta-studies are unreliable. They may pool studies that are not appropriate to pool. They may weight and combine studies that address different subpopulations without a precise definition of those subpopulations or knowledge of their proportion in the overall population. They may weight and combine studies that are not considered to be of equal reliability (e.g., because of methodological concerns over sample selection or measurement controls). The constructed weights are often subjective. So the resulting estimate of overall population mean does not have rigorous confidence intervals, and so is highly suspect. Many meta-studies are nothing more than numerical flimflam, designed to impress a naïve audience into believing that science was done with due diligence.

When you see a meta-study, think critically. In the popular media, meta-studies often boast sensational conclusions: saturated fat is not a concern; salt is not a concern; eggs are not a concern;

red meat is not a concern; a daily glass of red wine is good for you; coconut oil is good for you; aspartame is bad for you; cell phone use is bad for you; and living next to power lines is bad for you. In the past, there have been meta-studies with conclusions like: smoking doesn't cause lung cancer, asbestos doesn't pose a risk, and trans-fats are not harmful. It's important to realize that meta-studies often do not represent rigorous science.

Trying to combine related studies is a worthy goal as long as it can be done in a rigorous way. That's often not the case. Yet meta-studies and their publication proceed apace. For those looking to beef up their publication list, meta-analysis is a favored research strategy. After all, it's research on the cheap. You don't have to gather the data yourself; you don't even have to be an expert on the subject – you just cobble together existing studies and apply a few ad hoc maneuvers. Then you slap your name on it and there you have it: a low effort, quick, and inexpensive publication.

On a day-to-day basis, we frequently rely on casual meta-analysis to form opinions and make decisions. Often this leads to judgments based mostly on hearsay. In medicine, a doctor's opinions and decisions are shaped by med school training, personal experience, conversations with colleagues, journal articles, medical brochures, and inputs from drug and device reps. These are melded together in the doctor's mind in a loose, non-rigorous meta-analysis – again, one for which it's hard to attach meaningful accuracy and confidence.

Bias and bias compounded

Several kinds of bias commonly afflict data analysis and reporting. Among the most common are sample bias, publication bias, file drawer bias, and agenda-driven bias. *Sample bias* exists when a compelling argument can be made that the sample under study is not representative of the intended population. *Publication bias* refers to the tendency of journals to accept only the most sensational results, dismissing less exciting papers that may nevertheless contain useful information. *File drawer bias* is similar to publication bias, except that the authors themselves decide not to submit articles that they believe journals will reject as being too pedestrian. *Agenda-driven bias* is a catchall for several different kinds of bias – sample bias, study selection bias (in a meta-study), selective reporting, and exaggerated claims – that stem from the researcher's desire, or that of a patron, to promote a certain economic, social, personal, or political agenda.

When studies are cobbled together for a meta-study, the potential for bias is compounded: Not only might individual studies be biased, but the process of selecting the studies, or of selecting the committee members that select the studies, might also be biased.

Simpson's Paradox

Sometimes a trend that appears in different samples from a population reverses itself when the samples are pooled. Cases of this came to light over a century ago and were later branded as examples of *Simpson's Paradox*. Figure 9-5 shows a real-life medical example (from among other examples cited on Wikipedia).

Each entry in the table indicates the fraction of a test group who benefitted from the treatment. When looking at treatment performance on small stones and large stones separately, we see that Treatment A shows a higher success rate than Treatment B in both cases. So, one analysis might conclude that Treatment A is better than Treatment B. But a different analysis might pool the results from Treatment A, and pool the results from Treatment B, and compare – in which case Treatment B comes out ahead! A complete reversal!

What's going on here? One problem is with the pooling. To get a reliable estimate of a treatment's success rate in the greater population, you can't always just pool samples taken from different subpopulations. As mentioned above in the section on "Combining data", the success rates of the two samples associated with Treatment A must be combined as a weighted sum, reflecting the prevalence of small stones versus large stones in the overall population of individuals who have stones. Similarly for Treatment B.

	Treatment A	Treatment B
Small stones	*Group 1* 81/87 = 93%	*Group 2* 234/270 = 87%
Large stones	*Group 3* 192/263 = 73%	*Group 4* 55/80 = 69%
Both	273/350 = 78%	289/350 = 83%

Figure 9-5 *Test results from a real-life medical study on kidney stone treatment. The table indicates group success rates for two different treatments on two different stone sizes.*

Now if it should happen that small stones and large stones occur with equal prevalence, then the weights on the two samples are both 0.5, which gives the same answer as pooling. In this case, the numbers in Figure 9-5 represent an uncommon situation – it's not clear which analysis leads to the more reliable conclusion: the pooled analysis or the un-pooled. At least this much can be said: To some extent, when Simpson's Paradox occurs, it occurs because of discrepancies in the sample sizes. If the sample size for Treatment A was the same as for Treatment B, for each stone size, then Simpson's Paradox could not occur.

Subdividing data

In a meta-analysis, studies are combined with the goal of obtaining more reliable conclusions about an overall population. But it's also common to go in the other direction, in what might be called a *reverse meta-analysis*. We may start with a large random sample from a large population and compute its mean in order to estimate the population mean. Then we might consider various sub-samples of the sample in order to estimate the means of corresponding sub-populations, and see if there are significant differences among those means. Here are some examples:

- A new drug comes out and is widely prescribed. Over time, patients are seen to experience unforeseen harms or unforeseen benefits from the drug. The prevalence of these harms and benefits may be different for different groups of people based on gender, race, ethnicity, or other characteristics. These groups may warrant individual study.

- In 2009, the US Preventive Services Task Force (USPSTF) revised its 2002 guidelines for routine mammogram screening and now recommends that average-risk asymptomatic women begin regular screening at age 50 rather than age 40. The guidelines embody a "one-glove-fits-all" type of recommendation. On the other hand, a recent article titled, "Breast Cancer Statistics, 2015" in the journal *CA: A Cancer Journal for Clinicians*, reports that in the US, black women are more likely to be diagnosed with breast cancer at later stages of the condition than white women; breast cancer rates in black women are on the rise; black women die from breast cancer at a rate more than 40% higher than that for white women; and black women are more likely to be found with aggressive forms of the cancer. Certainly, these differences suggest that black women, as a subpopulation, warrant special study.

- Rates of cardiovascular disease in the US have been shown to vary significantly across different groups based on race, geography, lifestyle, and economic status. This represents a more useful understanding of cardiovascular disease than knowing just an overall national rate.

- Knowing the nationwide rate of melanoma in the US is not as useful as knowing the state-by-state rate of melanoma. For example, the rate in Colorado is considerably higher than that in Washington State, this being due to causal factors like altitude and sun exposure.

- There is a considerable difference in the rate of obesity from state to state in the US. Sure, you could quote the national rate. But that would mask differences in physical activity, diet preferences, and per capita income that might explain much of the state-by-state variation.

- The teen pregnancy rate is much higher in certain US states than in others – this is far more useful to know than just a national average. Such fact opens the door to investigating what is different about the high-rate states versus the low-rate states and using that information to try and remedy the problem.

Data dredging (fishing, snooping, mining)

Seek and ye shall find. Mathew 7:7

Data dredging – sounds like something you do when you don't have a clue as to what to do. Data dredging refers to testing many different hypotheses at the same time on the same set of data. It's also called *data fishing*, *data snooping*, and *data mining*.

Marketers dredge data to try and determine what consumer profile is likely to buy a certain product. Pollsters do it in the hopes of finding out what traits characterize a red voter versus a blue voter. The betting person wants to know what traits make a pony a winner. Data dredging is also used in science, finance, economics, and medicine. It has been used to implicate over a hundred genes in autism.

Given a random sample from a large population, and a large number of hypotheses to test, suppose we discover one that is satisfied by the sample. Can we say with high confidence that the hypothesis holds true for the population?

Frequently, no! If the number of hypotheses is large relative to the sample size, then the following can occur: With high probability, by chance alone, a random sample satisfies at least one of the hypotheses, but the population as a whole satisfies none of the hypotheses! So when data dredging finds an hypothesis that's true on the sample, we can't distinguish with high confidence whether this is a chance artifact of the sample or reflective of a truth in the larger population. The only way to resolve the issue is to see if the hypothesis holds up on a new random sample. Generally speaking, the probability of confirming the hypothesis on this second random sample is low unless the hypothesis is satisfied by the population.

Here are some examples:

The first involves what's called the *Law of Truly Large Numbers*, which says: Given a large enough number of observations, something outrageous is likely to occur by chance alone. For example, the chance of tossing a fair coin ten times and getting heads every time is about one in a thousand, not very likely. However, if 10,000 people play the game, the probability that they'll all be losers is a tad more than 0.0000452. In other words, with near certainty, there will be at least one person who tosses ten straight heads by chance alone. Should we credit such a person as being exceptionally gifted in the fine art of coin-flipping? No – because this observation cannot be separated from what we would have expected to occur by chance alone. Before awarding prizes, shouldn't we know, at least with high probability, that the winners are truly gifted? Shouldn't we test the winners again to see if they can repeat the feat that distinguished them from the pack – ten tosses, ten heads? For each winner, chances are roughly a thousand to one that the feat will be repeated.

The coin tossing example is similar to examples we see in the financial realm: Who is the exceptional investor? And in the sports realm: Who is the exceptional batter? But return in five years and the exceptional investor is an unheard of. Return in a year and the exceptional batter is a memory.

Another example of data dredging occurs when considering high-dimensional data and searching exhaustively to see if any pair of coordinates is "significantly correlated", meaning that knowledge of one coordinate value has predictive power in estimating another coordinate value. If the data points are k-dimensional, then there are roughly $(k \times k)/2$ coordinate pairs to consider, where each pair corresponds to an hypothesis of the form: "This coordinate is significantly correlated with that coordinate". Here's what can happen: A large population of k-dimensional data may satisfy none of these hypotheses, and yet, with high probability, a random sample that's not too large, will satisfy at least one of the hypotheses.

In one notorious example of data dredging, it was reported that increased coffee-drinking was correlated with increased rates of pancreatic cancer. The study was criticized for not following up with additional experiments to verify the link. In fact, later studies found no statistical support for the relationship, while some even suggested an inverse relationship.

Another example of data dredging occurs when we consider high-dimensional data that has one special coordinate and we are searching exhaustively to check if any of the other coordinates is "significantly correlated" with the special coordinate. For instance: Maybe all the coordinates are binary. Maybe the special coordinate represents whether a person has bought a certain product. Maybe each other coordinate represents whether the person possesses a certain trait. The data dredge is looking for traits that describe a person who is likely to buy the product.

Moral of the story: Data dredging is a legitimate way to identify potential hypotheses that are true of a large population.

But any such hypothesis should not be given credibility unless it has been validated on its own new random sample.

Cherry-picking by Big Pharma

Cherry-picking has been a common ploy of Big Pharma to get new drugs on the market and it shows little regard for public health. It's a practice designed to game the FDA's system for clearing new products. Here's how it works:

A company develops a new drug; then contracts out some number of independent clinical trials; then reports to the FDA only on those trials whose results show the drug in the best light. It's a total abuse of the vetting process, putting profits before health concerns. If it's not criminal, it should be. Let's look at this deception in more detail:

Suppose there are 10 independent trials, each with 400 participants randomly chosen from the target population. Individually, each trial's estimate of the drug's true success rate (the success rate in the target population) is within 5% accuracy at 95% confidence. But the probability that all the trial estimates are *simultaneously* within 5% of truth is only $(0.95)^{10} = 0.6 = 60\%$. (Each trial result is independent of the others, so it's like tossing a biased coin 10 times – the probabilities multiply.) Hence there is a significant chance that the highest trial result exceeds truth by more than 5%. So it cannot be claimed that the highest trial result is within 5% of truth at the 95% confidence level – to do so suggests the drug is better than it actually is. But that is exactly what drug companies do when they submit only their best trials to the FDA.

To honor the intention of the FDA's system for drug approval, what the pharmaceutical company should do is report the results of all 10 trials separately, together with all the relevant information about how they were conducted and any special concerns.

JEROME & SETH MALITZ

Ch. 10 Progress by Regression

In his autobiography, *Adventures of a Mathematician* (1991), Stanislaw Ulam recalls attending a lecture on physics. John von Neumann was sitting by his side. A slide projected on the screen showed a somewhat disheveled scatter of points. "Clearly," said the speaker, "the points lie on a line." Von Neumann leaned over to Ulam and whispered none too softly, "Well, at least it's clear they lie on a plane."

If image isn't everything in presenting data, it's often helpful in conveying its message. The speaker was trying to impress on the audience that the data was well-fit by a line, though Von Neumann wasn't buying it. In general, a curve or surface fitted to a collection of data points is considered an idealized representation of the data, not only clarifying its essential structure by smoothing out insignificant fluctuations, but also suggesting trends and possible dynamics that might have generated the data. Curve and surface fitting is common practice in economics, market analysis, business analysis, ecology, engineering, medical research, and many other areas.

These days, when electronic medical records can be mined from vast repositories like those maintained by the Veteran's Affairs Records Center and Kaiser Permanente (the latter with more than 11 million EMR's), a research project can examine a great many factors as possibly contributing to a given disease or condition, or affecting the performance of a given drug or therapy.

Representing each patient as a data point in a coordinate space, researchers might want to know how the value of a certain **output variable** (say longevity) relates to the values of one or more **input variables** or **factors** (say waist-to-hip ratio, sugar consumption, and blood pressure). When only one input variable is involved, a curve in two dimensions can be fitted to the data. When two input variables are involved, a surface in three dimensions can be fitted to the data. When several input variables are involved, it is no longer possible to depict a model fitted to the data – the three-dimensional space of everyday existence does not suffice. But mathematics can deal with spaces of any dimension, no matter how large – abstraction takes over where intuition leaves off.

Of course, the relationship between the output variable and an input variable could be studied separately for each input variable, but seeing how the output variable relates to the input variables *simultaneously* often provides much more information.

In a medical study involving many input variables, it is often important to isolate those that have the greatest predictive power in estimating the output variable. (As always, even if these input variables are highly predictive of the output variable, they do not necessarily have a causal influence on the output variable. Correlation is not necessarily causation. But a causal relationship might be there and it should be explored.) For example, the output variable might represent the severity of a disease, and the goal of the study might be to learn which are the most important factors contributing to the disease, in the hopes that practical ways exist to control those factors. But how do you determine which input variables have the strongest association with the output variable? When many input variables are being considered, this is not an easy question to answer and is one that still engages mathematicians and computer scientists today. When there are fewer input variables, or we're just considering small subsets of the input variables, the problem can be solved by a practical "brute force" method.

Fitting curves and surfaces to data points and quantifying the tightness and reliability of the fit is called **regression analysis** –

a peculiar name for a technique that is so often used to advance research. But whatever you call it, it's a powerful tool for gaining insight into the structure of data, suggesting patterns, trends, and causal relationships that may go well beyond your initial intuitions.

The model is the message

(variation on Marshall McLuhan)

Data is often messy – fluctuations may obscure an essential underlying structure or trend: Are the data points roughly arranged on a line (if 2D), or on a plane (if 3D), or in some other mathematically defined way? Regression analysis tries to find a comprehensible **model**, a curve or surface in this context, that describes the data with some level of fidelity.

In the simplest applications of regression analysis, the data points have two coordinates (x, y), where x is the input variable (also called the *independent* variable) and y is the output variable (also called the *dependent* variable). In this case, a model is a curve, interpreted as a predictor of y given x. Rarely is the predictor perfect.

Often, y is the sum of two parts: a part characterized by a formula on x, and a perturbation part that is either inessential or difficult to characterize. In engineering, the part of y described by the formula on x is commonly called the *signal*, while the perturbation part is called the *noise*. Perturbations often arise from unexplained ambient factors that affect the measurement of y, or from unexplained intrinsic factors within the measuring instrument itself.

The purpose of regression analysis is primarily to find a model that describes the signal in the data. The strategy is this: First select a family of curves or surfaces to consider; then select the model within that family that yields the tightest fit to the data. In two dimensions, the most common families are lines, parabolas, exponentials, and logarithms. In three dimensions, the most common families are planes and quadratics.

What is the right family of models to use when fitting a collection of data points? It depends on the application and purpose of the fit. As a rule, we look for the "simplest" type of model that meets our goals. If the goal is to highlight the most essential trend in the data, that may dictate one family of models. If the goal is to obtain the most accurate predictor of y versus x for values of x not used in the fit, a different family of models might be needed. In other cases, past experience or scientific theory may dictate the choice of model. In the next sections, we'll further discuss how to pick the right family of models, and the right model in the family,

An interesting example of a curve fit in medicine is the linear curve in Figure 10-1, which shows an approximate relationship between age and average *max heart rate*, in the general population. (Max heart rate is the highest heart rate a person can achieve during an exercise stress test without showing problems on an electrocardiogram. See "Heart rate" in Wikipedia.)

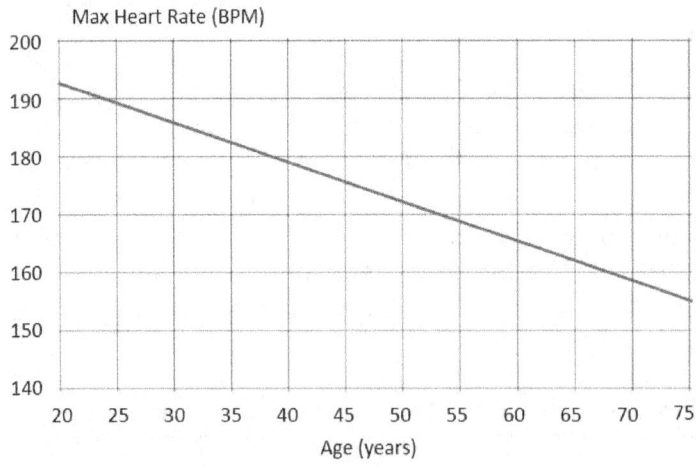

Figure 10-1 *The Robergs-Landwehr line is an approximate relationship between age and average max heart rate for that age.*

This curve is one of many that have been published by different research groups studying max heart rate. Most of these fitted curves are linear, but some are non-linear. (Again see the Wikipedia article.) However, they all point to an average decline of between 30 and 60 BPM over life. In Figure 10-1, it would be useful to see an "envelope" around the indicated line that captures, say, 90%, of people at each age. That would give a sense of the spread of max heart rate at each age. If a person's max heart rate is below the envelope, it may be indication of a problem.

The fitted curves in Figure 10-2 show approximate relationship between a girl's age and various percentiles of BMI. For example, the curve labeled "50%" indicates the approximate relationship between age and the 50th percentile of BMI for that age. (Google "BMI Graph Page Baylor School of Medicine".) The dots in the figure are the BMI readings of a particular individual at years 4, 6, 8, and 10. The upward drift of the dots across the curves suggest a weight-gain that may warrant attention.

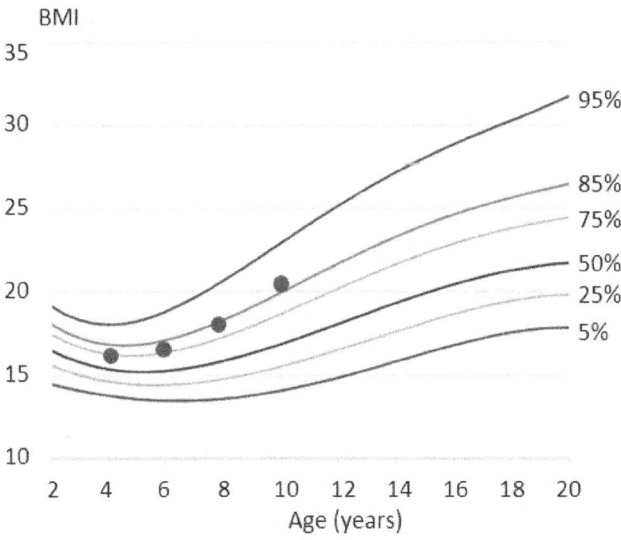

Figure 10-2 *Percentile curves showing the approximate relationship between a girl's age and various percentiles of BMI for that age. The four dots show a particular individual's readings over time.*

Other interesting curve fits that can be found online, show how average testosterone level varies with age in men, how average estrogen and progesterone levels vary with age in women, how average systolic and diastolic blood pressure varies with age, how risk of coronary heart disease varies with LDL (low-density lipoprotein) level in the blood, and how risk of all-cause mortality varies with resting heart rate.

Here are some other curve fits of interest, but we have not pursued whether they are available online: How does short term memory vary with age? How does associative memory vary with age? How does the ability to recognize geometric equivalence vary with age? Similar questions can be asked about reflexes, muscle strength, eyesight, hearing, and others.

A curve fitted to a given patient's measurements over time can predict what might be in store for that patient, and can advise on whether a medical intervention is necessary. In Figure 10-3, suppose the y-axis indicates a particular kind of measurement (e.g., blood pressure, white blood cell count, concentration of chemical or bacteria in the blood, etc.) and the x-axis indicates the times or dates at which measurements were taken. The leftmost figure shows a linear increase; the middle shows an exponential increase, and the rightmost shows a logarithmic increase. Seeing which trend is manifest by the data can be an important guide to doctor and patient as to the best course of action.

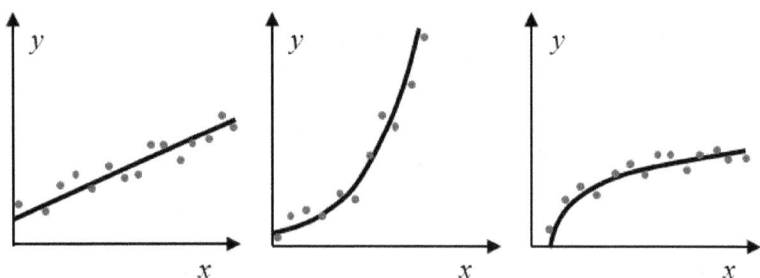

Figure 10-3 *From left to right: linear, exponential, and logarithmic curve fits to two-dimensional data sets. The y-axis represents the value of a measurement and the x-axis represents the date or time at which measurements were taken.*

In other applications, the data points have three coordinates, (x, y, z), where x and y are the input variables, and z is the output variable. In this case, the fitted model is a surface, interpreted as a predictor of z given x and y. Figure 10-4 shows a hypothetical fitted surface where the z-axis is risk of heart attack; the x-axis is blood pressure; and the y-axis is blood cholesterol level.

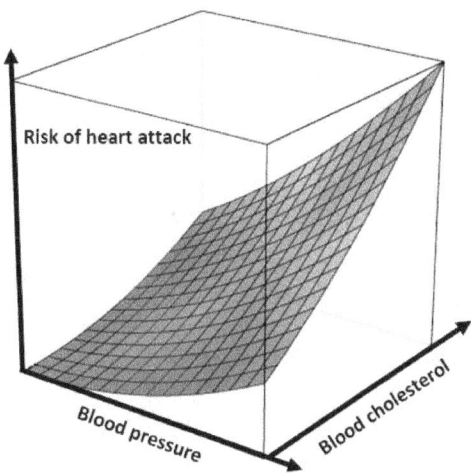

Figure 10-4 *Hypothetical fitted surface indicating how risk of heart attack varies with blood pressure and blood cholesterol.*

Additional applications involve more than three dimensions. In such cases, we can no longer visualize the data points or fitted surface, but we can still reason about them mathematically.

Getting the "best" fit from a family of models

Given a set of data points in two, three, or higher-dimensional space, and a family of models, which member in the family yields the "best" fit to the data? Within the family of lines, for example, there are infinitely many lines to choose from – which one is "best"?

To determine the best-fit model in a family of models, we first need a way of quantifying the **goodness-of-fit** of any model in the family relative to the data. One way to do this is to measure the positive vertical distance, called the **vertical residual**, from each data point to the model, and then take the average. (The vertical residuals are measured parallel to the axis of the output variable.) If $d_1, d_2,\ldots, d_n$ are the vertical residuals of n data points relative to a particular model, then the average residual, the value $(d_1 + d_2 +\ldots+ d_n) / n$, is a measure of the goodness-of-fit of that model. We might designate the best-fit model in the family to be the one that minimizes this average. See Figure 10-5.

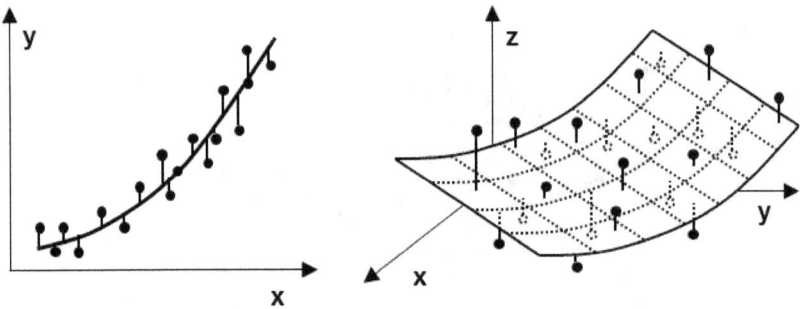

Figure 10-5 *Showing vertical residuals in two- and three-dimensional data relative to given models. At left, the output variable is y. At right, the output variable is z.*

However, with this notion of goodness-of-fit, there are generally an infinite number of models in the family that attain the minimum – that's a bit inconvenient. For this reason and others, the **best-fit model** in the family is usually taken as the one that minimizes the average (mean) *squared* residual, $(d_1^2 + d_2^2 + \ldots+ d_n^2) / n$. This is called the **least squares method** for best fit, and it has a *unique* solution, given by a mathematical formula. (It's somewhat advanced, so we won't give the formula here.)

In order to identify the best-fitting model in a family of models, we need a way of describing the models in that family.

For example, a general parabola has the form $y = ax^2 + bx + c$, where y is the output variable, a, b, and c are constants called *parameters*, and x is the input variable. So $y = 3x^2 + 5x - 4$ and $y = -2x^2 - 6x + 7$ are both parabolas, but with different parameters. Similarly, we might consider the family of lines $y = ax + b$, where a and b are the parameters of the line, a being the slope and b being the vertical axis intercept. Or we might consider the family of exponentials $y = ae^{bx}$, where again a and b are the parameters. If we're talking about surfaces, we might consider the family of planes $w = ax + by + cz + d$, where a, b, c, and d are the parameters, and x, y, and z are the input variables. In each case, once the family of models has been selected, the parameters of the best-fit member are found using the least squares method.

(*For the advanced reader*: Fitting two-dimensional data with a line or parabola is an instance of what's called *simple linear regression*. Fitting data of higher dimension with a plane or quadratic is an instance of what's called *multiple linear regression*. Linear regression refers to candidate models that are "linear in their parameters", but not necessarily "linear in their input variables".)

Just as the mean in one dimension is the point that minimizes the average squared distance to the data points, the best-fitting curve in a family of curves is the one that minimizes the average squared vertical distance to the data points. The average squared residual of the best-fit model is called the *mean squared error*, and is analogous to the notion of variance in one dimension. Its square root, the *root mean squared error*, is analogous to standard deviation. Once the best-fit model in the designated family has been identified, its goodness-of-fit measure is usually taken to be the root mean squared error.

Given an unbiased sample of data points from a large population, and the best-fit model (from a family of models) that has been fit to the sample, that model is an estimate of the best-fit model for the larger population. Mathematics tells us the confidence intervals, driven by sample size, that go with the estimated parameters of the best-fit model.

Getting the "right" family of models

Everything should be as simple as possible, but not more so.

Albert Einstein

Given a set of data points in two, three, or higher-dimensional space, what is the "right" family of models to use when fitting the data? The answer depends on the application and the purpose of the fit. In some cases, we may already know from existing theory or past experience what the right family of models is. In other cases, we may have to try out several different families and then compare the results of their best-fitting members, looking to strike the right balance between goodness-of-fit and the ability of the model to suppress unimportant fluctuations in the data. Sometimes, none of the families under consideration yields a good-enough fit for our purposes. In this case, we either have to relax the criterion for "good-enough", or entertain another family of models.

In practice, the most useful models are, as Einstein puts it, as simple as possible. Simpler models typically have fewer parameters and are less wiggly than more complex models. Although a complex model may fit the given data better than a simpler model, it usually doesn't emphasize the basic trend in the data as well, nor is it as good a predictor of y versus x for values of x not used in the fit. A model that fits the given data too tightly for an application is called an **over-fit**. A model that doesn't fit the given data tightly enough for an application is called an **under-fit**. In regression analysis, we're looking for the "sweet spot" – the right fit.

In Figure 10-6, we see a set of data points that has been fit by two curves from different families: a line (in black) and a "line plus sine wave" (in gray) which we'll denote by C. The curve C happens to come from a family that has four parameters. Its geometry is more complicated than that of the line, which comes from a family with two parameters. The data shows some amount of periodic fluctuation about the line fit, though the fluctuation appears relatively small. If the purpose of the fit is to suggest the most essential trend in the data, then the line might be considered a good fit, while the curve C is an over-fit. On the other hand, if the purpose of the fit is to obtain the most accurate predictor of y versus x for values of x not used in the fit, then curve C might be considered a good fit, while the line is an under-fit.

Does it make sense to look for a curve that fits the data even more tightly than C if we want the most accurate predictor of y versus x for values of x not used in the fit? No, not if the vertical residuals about curve C show "random" magnitudes, and they "average out to zero" when considering residuals above the curve as positive and below the curve as negative.

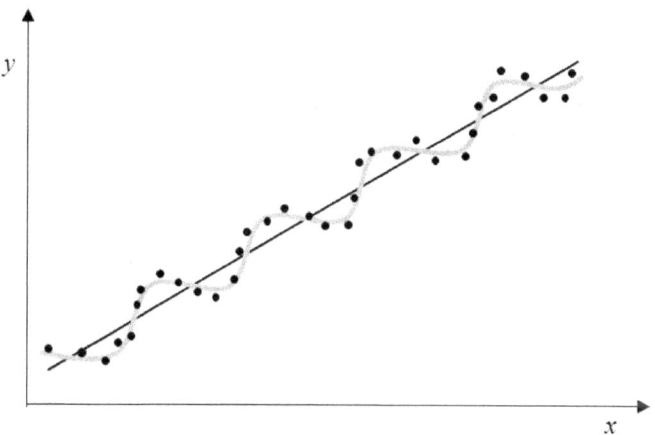

Figure 10-6 *Data fitted by a line (black) and a "line plus sine wave" (gray). The latter fit, though a better predictor of y versus x, may or may not be the preferred fit – it depends on the application.*

Figure 10-7 shows another set of data points that has been fit by two curves from different families: a line (in black) and a parabola (in gray). The parabola comes from a family that has three parameters. Its geometry is more complicated than that of the line, which comes from a family with two parameters. Clearly the line fit does not reflect the obvious down-then-up character of the data as we move from left to right along the x-axis. So the line might be considered an under-fit, while the parabola is considered a good fit.

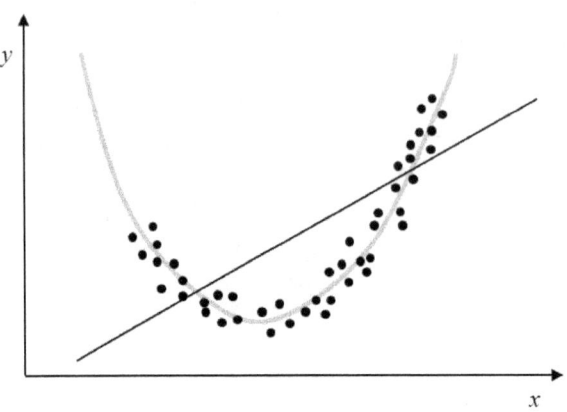

Figure 10-7 *A data set fitted by a line (black) and a parabola (gray). The line fit might be considered an under-fit because it doesn't register the "down-up" trend of the data as we move left to right.*

Our innate desire to find order within disorder often causes us to under-fit data. This happens, for example, when a model is fit to a subset of data that has been cherry-picked from a larger set, and the model is presented as a good fit for the larger set.

Fitting to a bar chart

Often a model is fit to a bar chart rather than to the original set of data points from which the bar chart was generated. In Figure 10-8 we see a hypothetical bar chart built from a collection of data points (x, y) (not shown), where x is the input variable and y is the output variable. The height of each bar is the average y-value of the data points whose x-values are in the corresponding bin. An artificial "top point" (not part of the original data set) has been introduced at the top of each bar. **Fitting to the bar chart** means fitting to these top points. In Figure 10-8 they have been fit by line.

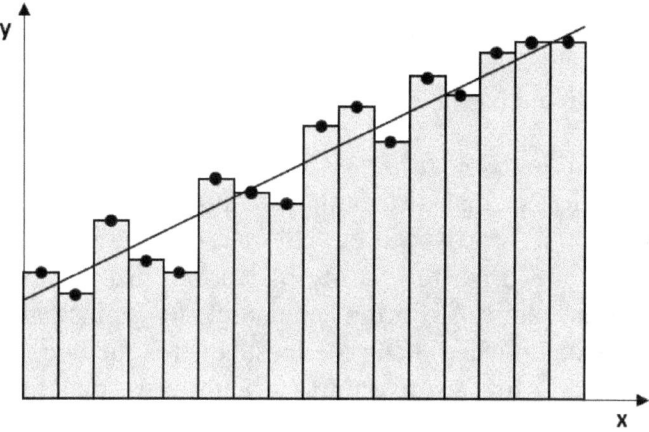

Figure 10-8 *A bar chart, its top points, and the line that best fits those top points (with respect to the least squares method).*

What if we were to fit the original set of data points by a line as well – how similar would the two fits be? Actually they can be very different depending on how even or uneven the distribution of data points is among the bins. For example, suppose the leftmost two bins each have a million data points, while the rest of the bins each contain only a hundred data points. Then in fitting a line to this data, the vast majority of residuals to be minimized are associated with the leftmost two bins. That means those bins exert much greater influence on the fit than the other bins, and so the resulting line will pass very close to their top points and slope downward from left to right. That's very different from the line shown in Figure 10-5. By contrast, if there were an equal number of data points per bin, then the resulting line fit would be identical to the one shown.

It's better to fit to the bar chart instead of to the original data if it's acceptable for the fit accuracy to be relaxed somewhat on dense bins in order to get better fit accuracy on sparse bins. But the fit should take into account that the mean y-value estimate of a sparse bin is less reliable (has larger confidence interval) than the mean *y*-value estimate of a dense bin, and hence a sparse bin should have less influence on the fit than a dense bin. This can be accomplished in a rigorous way by what's called the *weighted least squares method*. The resulting fit might be considered good if it can stay within, say, the 95% confidence interval associated with each observed bar height, or at least most bar heights.

Curve and surface fitting is also applied to probability histograms. The Normal distribution for IQ in Figure 7-1 is the result of such a fit. (Recall, a Normal distribution has two parameters μ and σ, so the family of Normal distributions is a two-parameter family.) Fitting a model to a histogram is sometimes accomplished using the least squares method, but for technical reasons, that's often not as straightforward as for other bar charts. (A more common technique is called *Maximum Likelihood Estimation*: Given a family of models such as the family of Normal distribution curves, this technique seeks the parameter values such that the observed histogram is "more likely to have come from" a model with these parameters than any other model in the family.)

Sometimes there is no good predictive model

In one dimension, the mean is not necessarily representative of the data – it depends on the dispersion of the data. If the dispersion is small, the mean is a good representative; if the dispersion is large, the mean is not a good representative. A similar issue arises when fitting models to two-, three-, and higher-dimensional data.

Both sets of data in Figure 10-9 show increasing vertical dispersion as we go from left to right. Hence any attempt at a curve fit to either set of data becomes an increasingly poor predictor of *y* versus *x* as we go from left to right.

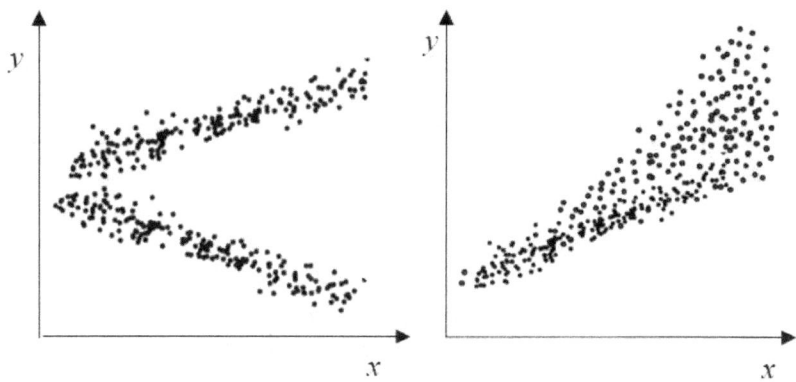

Figure 10-9 *Two sets of data that do not lend themselves well to a predictive curve fit: The data at left shows two distinct and divergent bands of density as you go from left to right. The data at right shows a strong increase in vertical dispersion as you go from left to right.*

The figure on the left suggests that the data should be viewed as coming from two different populations. This warrants investigation as to what characteristics (other than y value) underlie the difference between the two populations.

The most important factors

Not everything that can be counted counts, and not everything that counts can be counted.

Albert Einstein

When a number of factors are being considered simultaneously, we often want to know which are the most important for predicting the output variable. Regression analysis provides a rigorous framework for **factor reduction** – for identifying a smallest subset of factors that have the strongest association with the output variable, and for obtaining a model involving just those factors. This is useful for two reasons: (1) A model with fewer factors is easier to understand; (2) In a model with fewer factors, there are fewer causal links to explore in relation to the output variable, and so it becomes practical to think about controlling those factors as a means for controlling the output variable. For example, if the severity of a medical condition is tied to a number of factors, it may be impractical to try and address them all at once, but addressing a few of them, especially those that are the most significant, is both practical and sensible.

In general, the best-fit model (in a family of models) using *all* factors has better goodness-of-fit (smaller root mean squared error) than a best-fit model (in the same family) using only a subset of factors. In factor reduction, we're looking for a smallest subset of factors that does not sacrifice "too much" goodness-of-fit compared to the best-fit model using all the factors.

When a large number of factors are present at the start, optimal factor reduction can take an unacceptably long amount of time, so we may have to content ourselves with a less-than-optimal solution that yields a small subset, but not necessarily the smallest subset. However, when there are fewer than about 30 factors, there is a practical "brute force" algorithm that can get us the optimal solution: The algorithm explores all possible subsets of factors, proceeding smallest to largest, until a smallest subset is found such that the best-fit model satisfies the chosen threshold for goodness-of-fit. (Why is the algorithm not practical for more than 30 factors? If there are n factors to begin with, then there are as many as 2^n subsets to consider. If n exceeds 30, then 2^n exceeds a trillion, which is too many subsets for today's computers to handle in reasonable time.)

Similar to the concern in data dredging, a best-fit regression model that starts from many factors must be validated on a new random sample before it can be claimed with high confidence that it's a good fit on the larger population.

Interpolation and extrapolation

Prediction is difficult, especially about the future.

Niels Bohr

Suppose we want a curve that is a good predictor of a patient's blood pressure throughout the day. We might ask the patient to self-administer a blood pressure measurement once in the morning and once in the evening, and to do this over a period of several weeks. On the resulting data, we can perform a line fit. Each data point is a pair (x, y), where x is time of day, and y is, say, diastolic blood pressure. Half the points came from the morning and half from the evening. The constructed line fit is intended to predict not only morning and evening blood pressure, but blood pressure at any time of day in between. This is an example of what's called **interpolation** – we're using the fitted curve (in this case a line) to predict the value of y for values of x that are between the data points used in the fit, i.e., that are *inside* the range of x-values of the fitted data.

In the above example, the line will be a good predictor of blood pressure in the morning and evening, but it may not be a good predictor in the middle of the day, particularly for times that are far from the data points used to create the fit. Midday readings should be collected and compared to the fitted line's prediction. If the line is not a good predictor for these readings, then the new data should be added to the original data and a new curve fitted, perhaps using something other than a line.

Extrapolation uses a fitted model to make predictions *outside* the range of x-values of the fitted data. For example, if the input variable is time, and all the data points for the fit are contained within a particular interval of time, then applying the fitted model outside this interval, using it to make predictions about the past or future, is extrapolation. Models are extrapolated to predict weather, climate change, population growth, financial and economic trends, sports outcomes, and even the future of the universe. Other models take us back in time, to give us possible narratives on how and when creatures evolved, how climates and land masses changed, how cultures and languages spread, and how the universe came to be.

However, when we extrapolate a time-based model, whether into the future or past, we are making a big assumption: that the system dynamics posited for the present model will remain unaltered from present to future, or has remained unaltered from past to present.

However, depending on the context, some scientists doubt the validity of that assumption. Climatologists, for example, who try to predict climate far into the future, entertain the possibility of a catastrophic change in climate dynamics, a "tipping point," where the future does not behave like the past, where even an immediate worldwide adoption of green practices will no longer be sufficient to reverse or slow down the negative impacts of a changing climate. Many physicists today entertain the possibility that the current speed of light is different from what it was at an earlier time in the history of the universe – so much for "constants" of nature.

Other examples in history show how the dynamics of a situation, or our understanding of it, can change, and how models built on an earlier understanding can fail to have predictive power. In the 1960's, climatologists predicted that the world was entering a period of global cooling. These days the talk is all about global warming. In the same decade, M. King Hubbert famously predicted that worldwide "Peak Oil" would occur in the year 2000. Now it seems the world is awash in oil as well as other fossil fuels. Until 2006, almost everyone predicted that housing prices would just keep going up, up and up, and that our economy was in no danger of a precipitous collapse. Now we know better. Many believe, because of advances in medicine, that longevity in the US has been rising uniformly over the last thirty years, but in fact, there are places in the country where it has been declining. (See for example, "US life expectancy varies by more than 20 years from county to county", *Washington Post*, May 8, 2017.)

In trying to predict the future, we extrapolate models that have been verified on data from the present and near past. That's a reasonable thing to do. But we have to be cautious – extrapolation often does not come with a statistical guarantee of reliability.

The last statement applies to other examples. Time is not the only input variable on which a model might be extrapolated. For example, if a drug approved for use in adults (based on FDA clinical trials) is subsequently prescribed in off-label manner for children, and there is no statistical support for the practice, then this is an example of extrapolation – it extrapolates results for ages 18 and above into the range 18 and below. Similarly, it's an extrapolation if the drug is prescribed off-label for conditions other than those for which it was FDA-approved and for which no statistical evidence of efficacy and safety is available.

Curves as data points

Sometimes it's not just an isolated measurement that's of interest, but also the trend of the measurement over time.

Certainly, if a measurement is observed to be well outside the normal/healthy range, it may call for an immediate intervention. But even if the measurement is within the normal/healthy range, there may still be reason for concern if the trend described by this and past measurements is unfavorable. Examples of measurements where trends are important to watch: blood pressure; percent of time in A-fib; white blood cell count; level of a chemical in the blood; pulse rate; and so on.

To characterize the trend of a patient's measurements, we need to fit the data with a curve (from an appropriate family of curves), as shown in Figure 10-10. Once we have the curve, the question arises: Does it represent an acceptable trend or does it call for an immediate attention?

This question is simplified by representing curves themselves as data points: For example, a fitted line $y = ax + b$, where a and

b are parameter values, can be represented by the 2-dimensional point (a, b). Or maybe we only care about the line's slope a, which can be represented by a 1-dimensional point. A fitted parabola $y = ax^2 + bx + c$, where a, b, and c are parameter values, can be represented by the 3-dimensional point (a, b, c). Or maybe we only care about the a and b terms of the parabola, in which case the representation is just the 2-dimensional point (a, b).

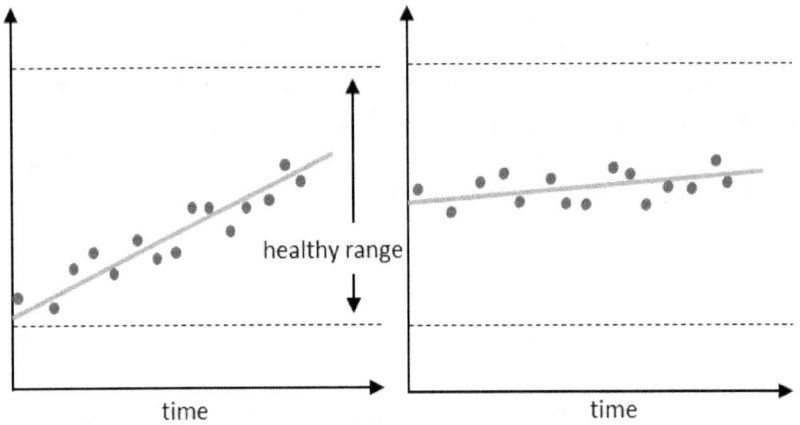

Figure 10-10 *In both diagrams, the patient's measurement readings are in the healthy range. But the trend line for the patient on the left is very steep, suggesting a problem that needs immediate attention.*

Given a linear trend, characterized as a 2-dimensional data point (a, b), how do we determine if the patient's condition warrants immediate attention? Given a parabolic trend, characterized as a 3-dimensional data point (a, b, c), how do we determine if the patient's condition warrants immediate attention?

These are question about how to determine appropriate cutoff boundaries in two, three, and higher dimensions. Even in one dimension, it's a question: How do we determine the appropriate cutoff value for deciding if the patient's condition warrants immediate action? These questions are addressed in the next two sections.

(*Note: The next two sections are somewhat more complicated than previous material. The reader can choose to skip these sections without loss of continuity.*)

Getting the best cutoff value

Suppose a continuous measurement x (e.g., blood calcium level) is used to determine whether or not a patient has a certain disease that warrants medical attention. If x^* is a candidate *cutoff value* for x, then a test $T(x^*)$ for the disease might return test positive if $x > x^*$, and test negative otherwise. Suppose there is a gold standard test D for the disease, but it is not the preferred method of diagnosis. (It may be that test D is not timely enough, or is too invasive, uncomfortable, inconvenient, or expensive.) What is the best choice of cutoff value x^* such that the test $T(x^*)$ most closely matches the gold standard in the general population?

A sensible answer is to get the value of x^* that minimizes the total error probability, $P(T(x^*) \cap \tilde{D}) + P(\tilde{T}(x^*) \cap D)$, that we saw in Chapter 8 (section "Conditional probability").

Suppose that for the sake of study, there is an available sample of patients from a population of interest who have received the gold standard test, half showing D positive and half showing D negative, each half itself an unbiased sample of its kind. Let's see how this sample can be used to estimate the desired value x^*:

For any value of x, let $P(D|x)$ denote the conditional probability (in the general population) that a person has the disease given that the person's measurement value is "near" x. Without going into detail, we can estimate $P(D|x)$ using the provided sample, Bayes' Formula, and an estimate of the disease prevalence $P(D)$ in the general population. After estimating $P(D|x)$ for various values of x, we can fit those values with a curve. This fitted *disease risk curve,* which we'll denote, $f(x)$, estimates $P(D|x)$ for each value of x. If $f(x)$ increases as x increases, then it can be shown (using the calculus) that the value of x^* that minimizes the total error probability occurs where

$f(x^*)$ equals ½. (If instead, the goal was to find the value of x^* that minimizes a total weighted error, where a is the penalty for a false positive and b is the penalty for a false negative, then the x^* we seek occurs where $f(x^*)$ equals $a/(a+b)$.)

In some applications, the test $T(x^*)$ is not intended as a replacement for the gold standard test, but rather as a preliminary screen to determine if the gold standard should be applied (e.g., screen the patient to decide if a biopsy or imaging procedure is recommended). Specifically, if the screening test $T(x^*)$ comes up positive, then apply the gold standard; otherwise do not. In this scenario, what is the best cutoff value x^* to use in the test $T(x^*)$? Again, a sensible answer is to identify the value of x^* that minimizes the total error probability or total weighted error. (In the latter, the penalty for a false positive is the penalty for an unnecessary application of the gold standard test, and the penalty for a false negative is the penalty for missing the disease entirely.)

What if test $T(x^*)$ is itself the gold standard test, meaning that there is no other independent gold standard test to compare against? For example, measurement of blood pressure is the sole test used to make a diagnosis of hypertension. What is the best choice of cutoff value x^* in this situation? A sensible answer is to choose the cutoff value x^* such that, on an historical set of patients, the average net benefit of intervention for patients slightly above x^* is equal to the average net benefit of no intervention for patients slightly below x^*.

Imagine two curve fits on the sample of historical patients: One curve fit estimates, for each value of x, the average net benefit experienced by patients whose measurement was x at the time of intervention. The other curve fit estimates, for each value of x, the average net benefit experienced by patients whose last measurement was x and did not receive the intervention. The cutoff x^* mentioned above is where the two curves cross.

It's important to recognize that the optimal cutoff value might vary depending on the population being considered. It may not be justified to use the same cutoff value for all populations.

Getting the best cutoff boundary

Sometimes several different continuous measurements are assessed at the same time to determine if the patient has a certain disease, or for use as a screening tool to decide whether or not a gold standard test should be applied. For example, in Chapter 3 (section "Visit to the dermatologist"), we mentioned the "ABCDE method" for deciding whether a skin mole should be biopsied for melanoma – biopsy being considered the gold standard for melanoma. Here the screening method requires that a dermatologist visually inspect the mole to assess its degrees of: **A**symmetry, **B**orders (irregularity), **C**olor (variegation), **D**iameter, and **E**volution (of size, shape, and color, over time), and then come to a decision.

But a dermatologist's evaluation of such features is often imprecise and subjective, which effects the rigor of the decision-making. A computer on the other hand, equipped with special-purpose image processing algorithms, can quantify such features in a precise and objective way, and rigorously determine whether or not a biopsy is warranted.

At the highest level, here's how an automated screening method for melanoma might work: First, it precisely measures (A, B, C, D, E) for the mole and interprets the result as a point in 5-dimensional space. Then, depending on which side of a particular *cutoff boundary* (*cutoff surface*) the point resides, the automation recommends biopsy or no biopsy. So, what is this cutoff boundary? How is it obtained?

For ease of discussion, let's consider a 2-dimensional analogy to the above question. Suppose there are just two continuous measurements, x and y, that will be used to decide whether or not a patient has a certain disease. If c^* is a *cutoff curve* in the xy-plane, then a test $T(c^*)$ for the disease might return test positive if the patient's measurement point (x, y) is on one side of the curve c^*, and test negative on the other. Suppose there is a gold standard test D for the disease. What is the best choice of cutoff curve c^* such that test $T(c^*)$ most closely matches the gold standard D in the general population?

A sensible answer is to look for the curve c^* that minimizes the total error probability, $P(T(c^*) \cap \tilde{D}) + P(\tilde{T}(c^*) \cap D)$. This curve c^* can be estimated in similar way to the previous section:

Again, suppose there is an available sample of patients from a population of interest who have received the gold standard test, half showing D positive and half showing D negative, each half itself an unbiased sample of its kind. For any pair of measurement values (x, y), let $P(D|x,y)$ denote the conditional probability (in the general population) that a person has the disease given that the person's measurement values are "near" (x, y). Let $f(x,y)$ denote a *disease risk surface* that estimates $P(D|x,y)$ for each pair of values (x, y). This surface can be constructed from the provided sample. Suppose that $f(x,y)$ increases as either x or y increases.

To simplify the discussion, suppose that the surface $f(x,y)$ is the inclined plane (gray) shown in Figure 10-11. Consider a horizontal plane (also shown) slicing through the surface $f(x,y)$ at some height (i.e., risk level for the disease) z above the xy-plane. Then the intersection of the two surfaces is a curve (in this case a line) all of whose points are at height z. Project this curve down to the xy-plane and let $c(z)$ denote the resulting curve, called a *level curve*. Again, all points (x, y) on the curve $c(z)$ have the same risk level z.

Whatever curve c^* minimizes the total error probability, it doesn't make sense that it would separate points (x, y) that are at the same risk level – points with the same risk level should stay together one side of c^* or the other. It follows that the optimal curve c^* takes the form of a level curve $c(z^*)$ for some optimal cutoff value z^*. So the problem here boils down to finding the value of z^* that minimizes the total error probability, namely $P(T(c(z^*)) \cap \tilde{D}) + P(\tilde{T}(c(z^*)) \cap D)$. It can be shown (using the calculus) that this value of z^* equals ½. (If instead, the goal was to find the value of z^* that minimizes a total weighted error, where a is the penalty for a false positive and b is the penalty for a false negative, then the z^* we seek is $a/(a+b)$.)

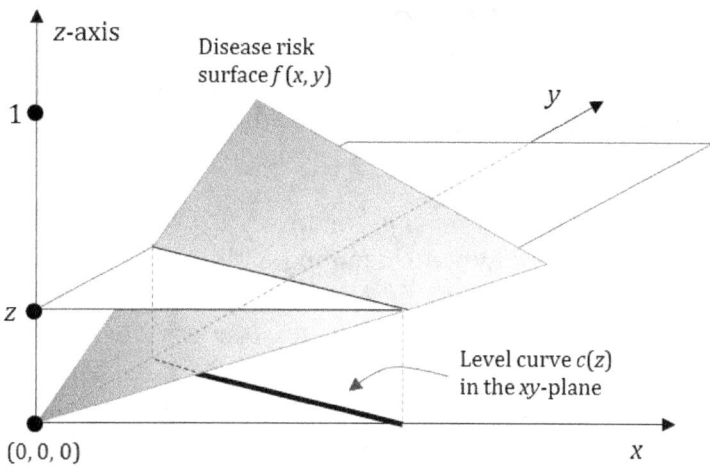

Figure 10-11 *Showing the level curve c(z) formed by intersecting the disease risk surface f(x, y) with a horizontal plane of height z, and projecting down to the xy-plane.*

Note that we don't explicitly need the cutoff curve $c(z^*)$ in order to know which side of the curve a query point (x, y) resides on: all we need to know is z^*. The query point is on one side of the curve if $f(x,y)$ is greater than z^*; on the other side if it is less than z^*.

When more than two continuous measurements are involved in the test T, everything we've done here for two dimensions can be generalized to higher dimensions.

For example, a disease risk surface $f(A,B,C,D,E)$ can be constructed in six-dimensional space that estimates the risk that a skin mole with measurement values (A,B,C,D,E) is melanoma.

In fact, over the last few years, a number of skin cancer apps (e.g., SkinVision) have been developed for smart phones. Once the user enters the app and takes a photo of the skin mole, the app computes rigorous, precise, objective measures of A, B, C, and D. If the user photographs the mole at different points in time, the app is able to compute a rigorous, objective measure of E. The app then makes a decision: recommend biopsy or no biopsy. Some manufacturers claim their apps are as good as the average dermatologist in deciding whether or not a biopsy is warranted. We do not know if those claims are credible at present. But eventually they will be.

Automation will eventually improve the reliability of the biopsy analysis itself. When examining a skin tissue sample for melanoma, the lab is looking for telltale signs of the disease, such as atypical distributions of melanocytes (the melanin-producing cells of the skin). But how atypical is atypical? Again, when humans evaluate such things, the answer tends to be subjective and imprecise. But computerized image processing algorithms will be able to provide answers that are objective and precise.

What if test $T(c^*)$ is itself the gold standard test for deciding whether or not an intervention is warranted, meaning that there is no other independent gold standard test to compare against? What is the best choice of cutoff boundary c^* in this situation? Similar to what was said in the previous section concerning a single measurement, the boundary c^* should be defined such that, on an historical sample of patients, the average net benefit of intervention for patients slightly on one side of c^* is equal to the average net benefit of no intervention for patients slightly on the other side of c^*.

It's important to recognize that the optimal cutoff boundary might vary depending on the population being considered. It may not be justified to use the same cutoff boundary for all populations.

Ch. 11 Decisions, Decisions, Decisions

Don't just do something. Stand there.

Anonymous

Which treatment is best? Is it better to do nothing rather than something? Should I get on this drug? Should I get vaccinated? Is it better to medicate or operate? Is it better to treat with intent to cure or intent to control? The answer: it depends. It can depend on the age, gender, build, or race of the patient, the patient's overall state of health and medical history, the severity of the symptoms, and of course, the patient's goals, and possibly even the time and money the patient can spend on treatment and recovery. But it shouldn't depend on the mindset, training, or practice style of the physician.

When minor ills and injuries occur – insect bite, headache, stomachache, diarrhea or constipation – treatment is often not controversial and can be found in the bathroom medicine cabinet, a veritable apothecary replete with creams and ointments, plasters and patches, pills and capsules.

But in other cases, the condition that requires treatment is more serious, and there may be several actions to choose from. Devoting more thought to treatment selection may significantly improve the chances of a good outcome.

But often, a treatment that might benefit the patient in some ways, can potentially harm the patient in others. So, when deciding among treatments, it's useful to compare them based on the odds of being helped, the odds of being harmed, and meaningful guarantees on how well those odds are known. This information can be obtained from rigorous statistics on samples of historical patients like the current patient. The results can be expressed in convenient ways that can serve as patient decision aids, aids that can help patients identify which treatments are most likely to meet their goals. Among notable decision aids: treatment success rate, ARR, ARI, histograms of benefit and harm, and diagrams called decision trees.

Is it safe? Is it effective?

But how are safety and efficacy determined? By using rigorous statistics. For example, here's a way of estimating the efficacy of a vaccine for a disease:

Select an unbiased sample E from the population of vaccinated individuals and call this the **experimental group**. Select an unbiased sample C from the population of unvaccinated individuals and call this the **control group**. Let p_E denote the fraction of individuals in E who developed the disease. Let p_C denote the fraction of individuals in C who developed the disease. Then p_E and p_C are estimates of the disease rates in the vaccinated and unvaccinated populations. Loosely speaking, the smaller p_E versus p_C, the more effective the vaccine.

Suppose p_C is 11% with 95% confidence interval [9%, 13%]. Suppose p_E is 6% with 95% confidence interval [4%, 8%]. The estimated risk reduction (in getting the disease) associated with the vaccine is then 11% − 6% = 4%. With confidence of at least 0.95 times 0.95, or about 90%, the vaccine's risk reduction for the general population is between 9% − 8% = 1% and 13% − 4% = 9%. So, the estimated risk reduction has a 90% confidence interval of [1%, 9%]. (In fact, a more sophisticated mathematical argument gives a smaller 90% confidence interval, but we won't dwell on that here.)

In practice, **vaccine effectiveness** is usually estimated as $(p_C - p_E)/p_C$, or equivalently, $1 - (p_E/p_C)$, and comes with a confidence interval that depends on the sample sizes. If the sample sizes are large, and the ratio p_E/p_C is small, then we can say with high confidence that the vaccine's effectiveness for the general population is high.

Given the numbers above, the estimated vaccine effectiveness is $1 - (6\% / 11\%) = 55\%$. With confidence of at least 0.95 times 0.95, or about 90%, the vaccine's effectiveness for the general population is between $1 - (8\% / 9\%) = 12\%$ and $1 - (4\% / 13\%) = 70\%$. So, the estimated effectiveness has (an asymmetric) 90% confidence interval of [12%, 70%]. (Again, a more sophisticated mathematical argument gives a smaller 90% confidence interval, but we won't get into that here.)

Based on large amounts of historical data, the estimated effectiveness of polio vaccine is nearly 100%, with nearly 100% confidence. By contrast, the annual flu vaccines from 2008 to 2017 each had an estimated effectiveness in the range 40% to 60%, barring the outliers of 2015 and 2017 where the estimated effectiveness was only 19% and 10%, respectively. All of these estimates have 95% confidence intervals of about plus-minus 7%.

The question of safety is addressed in a similar way to efficacy. For example, when exploring the safety of a vaccine, we compare the rate of a particular harm in the experimental (vaccinated) group E with the rate of that harm in the control (unvaccinated) group C. Loosely speaking, the larger the harm rate in E versus the harm rate in C, the less safe is the vaccine. The vaccines for polio, tuberculosis, tetanus, measles, mumps, rubella, chicken pox, and HPV are among vaccines that are considered to be exceedingly safe.

What's described above is essentially the same process that a drug company has to follow in order to get FDA approval for a new drug: Certain standards of efficacy and safety have to be demonstrated in clinical trials, where the results of an experimental group (those given the drug) are compared with the results of a control group (those not given the drug). It has to be demonstrated, with high confidence, that the drug is at least somewhat effective and not catastrophically unsafe.

ARR, RRR, and NNT

Suppose we're told about a drug that reduces the risk of an adverse health event (e.g., heart attack, stroke). The efficacy of such a drug is usually expressed in one of two ways – as ARR or RRR:

In a typical drug study, there is an experimental group E (an unbiased sample of people who were given the drug) and a control group C (an unbiased sample of people who were not given the drug). Let p_E denote the fraction of people in the experimental group who eventually suffered the adverse event. Let p_C denote the fraction of people in the control group who eventually suffered the adverse event. For instance, maybe p_C equals 4/1000 and p_E equals 1/1000. Then $p_C - p_E = 3/1000 = 0.3\%$ is an estimate of the drug's **Absolute Risk Reduction** (ARR) for the general population, and it comes with a confidence interval that depends on the sample sizes. The drug's ARR is the probability that the drug will prevent you from suffering the event – the probability that you will actually benefit from the drug.

Dividing ARR by p_C gives the ratio $(p_C - p_E)/p_C$, which is an estimate of the drug's **Relative Risk Reduction** (RRR) , and it also comes with a confidence interval that depends on the sample sizes. In our current example, the drug's RRR is estimated as 3/1000 divided by 4/1000, which equals 3/4 or 75%. Notice that vaccine effectiveness, mentioned in the previous section, is also expressed as a relative risk reduction.

Since p_C is usually less than one, RRR is at least as large as ARR – often a lot larger – and so sounds more impressive. In advertising, RRR is often used in place of ARR to give the impression that a drug is more likely to be beneficial than it actually is. Of the two numbers, the ARR is the one that patients and doctors should really care about, especially given that most drugs present risks for harmful side effects and some drugs incur significant out-of-pocket costs. It's okay to go by RRR if the condition being addressed is of serious concern and the risk of harmful side effects and cost of the drug are minimal. That is why vaccine effectiveness is usually expressed as RRR.

Taking the reciprocal of ARR, in other words computing 1/ARR, we get the drug's **Number Needed to Treat** (NNT). In our current example, NNT is estimated at 1000/3, or about 333. The interpretation is that about 333 people have to take the drug in order for one person to benefit from it. In general, the smaller the NNT, the more likely a patient will benefit from the drug. The ideal NNT is 1, where every individual who takes the drug benefits from it. NNT is generally thought to be an easier concept for people to understand than ARR (the latter expressing a probability).

Although NNT is frequently cited, it's usually not provided with a confidence interval, and that's a fault.

Similar to NNT, the **Number Needed to Screen** (NNS) is used to characterize the quality of a health screening test — it estimates the number of people who must undergo the test (and who will receive treatment if test positive) in order for one person to benefit from the test. The estimate should be provided with a confidence interval. Examples of tests for which NNS numbers are available include the regular PSA screening testing for prostate cancer and the regular mammogram screening test.

When estimating the risk of a particular harm associated with exposure to a drug or substance, the numbers of interest are **Absolute Risk Increase** (ARI), **Relative Risk Increase** (RRI), and **Number Needed to Harm** (NNH), which are defined similarly to ARR, RRR, and NNT. In particular, the ARI is estimated as $p_E - p_C$, where p_E is the fraction of people in the experimental (exposure) group E who exhibited the harm, and p_C

is the fraction of people in the control (non-exposure) group C who exhibited the harm. Again, these estimates should be provided with confidence intervals.

It can sometimes be tricky to decide between two or more drugs based on their ARR's. For example, one drug might have an ARR of 40% with a 95% confidence interval of [39%, 41%], while the other drug has a higher ARR of 45% but a wider 95% confidence interval of [35%, 55%]. Which drug is better? Unfortunately, the statistics don't make the choice clear in this case, but do indicate the need for further studies using larger samples and hence delivering tighter confidence intervals.

When a drug is intended to relieve a chronic symptom or cure a condition that will not otherwise go away on its own, we can talk about the **success rate** of the drug, which is estimated as the fraction of individuals in an experimental group (of people who are taking the drug) who experience the desired effect of the drug. Again the estimate is useful only if accompanied by a confidence interval.

Let's look at a couple of real-world examples that involve some of the numbers introduced above:

According to the article, "Statin-related adverse events: a meta-analysis", *Clinical Therapeutics*, Jan. 2006, the treatment of cardiovascular disease with statin drugs had an estimated NNT of about 30 for the population of at risk patients. When considering potential serious harms caused by the drug, the NNH is about 3400. This paper suggests that patients at risk for cardiovascular disease are much more likely to be helped by a statin drug than harmed by it.

In the October 2015 issue of *The Lancet*, WHO published a large study that concluded there is an 18% increased risk of colorectal cancer per 50g of processed red meat eaten per day. That's 18% per hot dog. That sounds like a big, scary number, but let's put it in perspective: WHO is saying that the estimated RRI for colorectal cancer due to eating a hot dog a day is 18%, which is to say that $(p_E - p_C)/p_C$ is about 18%. Here p_E is the risk of developing colorectal cancer in people who eat a hot dog a day, and p_C is the risk of developing colorectal cancer in people who don't eat red meat. In the US, the lifetime risk of colorectal cancer is about 5% (this includes people who eat red meat and those who don't.) So p_C is at most 5%. Now the estimated ARI for colorectal cancer due to eating a hot dog a day is $p_E - p_C$, which we recognize as the RRI times p_C, which according to WHO, is at most 0.18 times 0.05, which is less than 1%. So, the lifetime risk of getting colorectal cancer as a direct result of eating a hot dog a day is less than 1%.

Histograms of benefits and harms

Often it makes more sense to ask, "What level of benefit (or harm) might I get from this treatment?", rather than, "Could this treatment benefit (or harm) me?". Here, a useful decision aid is a *benefit* (or *harm*) *histogram* built from a sample of historical patients, showing the fraction of patients who experienced each level of benefit (harm). A "confidence envelope", the histogram equivalent of a confidence interval, should be provided with the histogram. The larger the sample, the more accurately the histogram approximates what's would happen in the larger population.

Such histograms may be used to show the distribution of patient experience for things like pain, strength, mobility, implant lifetime, recovery time, recurrence time, and overall patient satisfaction.

Suppose we're comparing two benefit histograms, one for treatment *A* and the other for treatment *B*. Suppose both histograms are reliable estimates of what would happen in the larger population. Is it easy to determine which histogram (treatment) is better? Answer: sometimes yes; sometimes no.

If for any benefit level *x* (let's assume larger *x* means greater benefit), the amount of area (probability) to the right of *x* within histogram *B* is at least as large as the amount of area (probability) to the right of *x* within histogram *A*, then *B* is clearly at least as good as *A*. But if this kind of relationship does not exist between the two histograms, the question as to which histogram (treatment) is better is not always clear-cut. Different patients may have different opinions.

A common way of choosing between benefit histograms *A* and *B* is to prefer the one with the larger mean. But what if *B* has larger mean than *A* and also larger standard deviation than *A*? See Figure 11-1. With this information alone, it's not clear which is the better histogram.

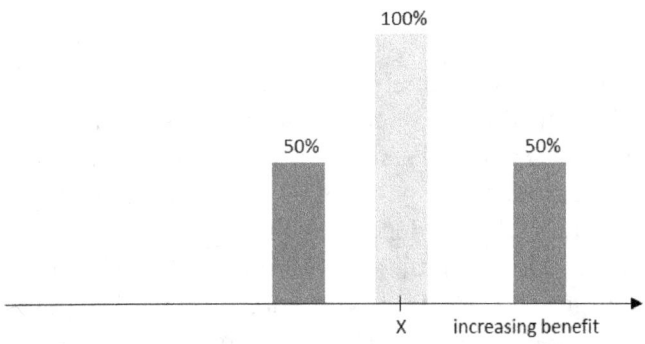

Figure 11-1 *Benefit histogram A (light) shows that 100% of patients obtain benefit level X. Its mean is X and its standard deviation is zero. Benefit histogram B (dark) shows a 50-50 split. Its mean is a little above X, but its standard deviation is greater than zero. Which histogram (treatment) is better?*

Even if *B* has larger mean than *A* and smaller standard deviation than *A*, the decision can still be tricky. See Figure 11-2.

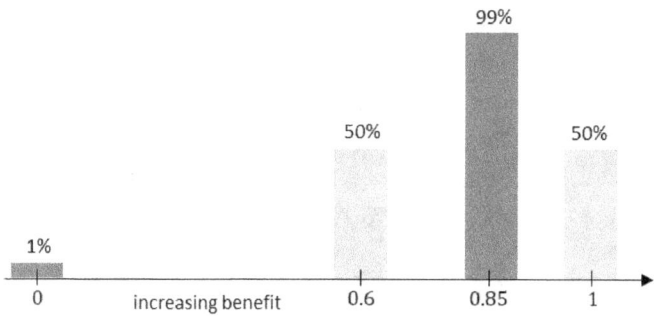

Figure 11-2 *Benefit histogram A (light) has mean 0.8 and standard deviation 0.2. Benefit histogram B (dark) has mean 0.84 and standard deviation 0.084. Which histogram (treatment) is better?*

Another possible way of choosing between A and B is to prefer the one that is more likely to deliver the higher benefit. But consider the example in Figure 11-3. Your chances of getting a better outcome from B compared to A are 60%, but it's questionable whether B should be considered better than A.

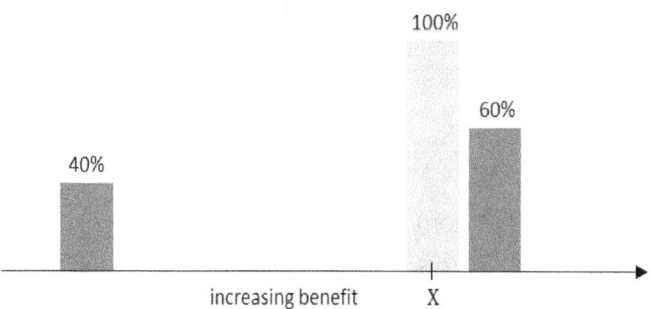

Figure 11-3 *Benefit histogram A (light) shows that 100% of patients get benefit level X. Benefit histogram B (dark) shows that 60% of patients get benefit level higher than X, while 40% get benefit level much lower than X. Which histogram (treatment) is better?*

Here's another thing that can happen: Given benefit histograms A, B, C, let's define "A is better than B" to mean that A is more likely to deliver higher benefit than B. Then the following can occur: A is better than B; B is better than C; and C is better than A! In other words, for any histogram among A, B, C, that you might pick, there's a better one you could have picked! Can this actually happen? Yes. This was considered so strange in 1950 that it came to be known as *Arrow's Paradox*, after Kenneth Arrow (recipient of the 1971 Nobel Prize in economics) who first observed it. Here's a concrete example:

Suppose histogram A has three bars located at values 3, 4, 8, each with probability 1/3. Suppose B has three bars located at values 2, 6, 7, each with probability 1/3. Suppose C has three bars located at values 1, 5, 9, each with probability 1/3. Each histogram is like that of a fair "three-sided die". The mean of each histogram is 5. So comparing the histograms by their means tells us nothing. But you can verify (similar analysis as was used for the game of craps in Example 3 of Chapter 7) that 5/9 of the time a random toss from A will be larger than a random toss from B; 5/9 of the time a random toss from B will be larger than a random toss from C; and 5/9 of the time a random toss from C will be larger than a random toss from A. So A is better than B; B is better than C; and C is better than A. In this case, there is nothing to recommend one histogram (treatment) over any other.

Were you satisfied with your treatment?

Often, multiple criteria come into play when comparing treatments. Trying to be evidence-based about things, one might wonder if it isn't enough to ask just one question of historical patients, "Were you satisfied with your treatment?", and then pick the treatment with the highest percentage of "yes" responses? Unfortunately, there are several downsides to this approach: First, the question doesn't account for timeframe – patients may respond differently when queried one year after treatment versus five years after treatment. Second, it's reasonable to question whether the prior patients are similar enough to the current patient in terms of their standards for satisfaction. Third, prior patients might say they were satisfied with their treatment, being unaware that a different treatment would likely have delivered an even better result.

Decision trees

Sometimes a decision we make now can lead to one of several possible outcomes, some of which may necessitate other decisions later. Patients should understand the possible outcomes associated with each treatment and the choices they might face in the future. This is true for patients contemplating joint replacement surgery, neck or back surgery, hand or wrist surgery, bariatric surgery, cancer surgery, cosmetic surgery, and many more. It's true for patients who are considering treatment with intent to cure versus treatment with intent to control. Patients need to know what could be in store for them, and need to be in position to ask the right questions to help them identify the best treatment. A tree-like diagram called a **decision tree** can help.

The decision tree in Figure 11-4 is adapted from a teaching example in the article, "Uncertainty and Decisions in Medical Informatics", *Methods Inf Med,* Mar. 1995. It shows the decisions and chance outcomes faced by a patient who arrives to the clinic with a badly infected foot that has turned gangrenous. The tree is ordered from left to right. The leftmost node corresponds to the first decision that the patient must make: antibiotics or below knee amputation (BKA). The antibiotics route might be successful and lead to full recovery, or it might lead to a worsening situation where the patient faces a second choice: more aggressive antibiotic treatment or above knee amputation (AKA).

In a decision tree, there are *decision nodes* (also called *action nodes*), as well as *chance nodes* and *leaf nodes*. Each decision (action) node is indicated by a square and originates one or more action branches. The leftmost decision node is called the *root node*. Each chance node is indicated by a circle and originates two or more chance branches representing different chance outcomes. Each leaf is indicated by a triangle and represents a terminus in the modeling. A root-to-leaf path represents a possible medical trajectory of the patient. In general, a branch out of a decision node can feed into another decision node, a chance node, or a leaf. Similarly, for a chance node. The number of action branches out of the root may number more than two. The branches emerging from a node are *exclusive* and *exhaustive* – meaning a patient cannot traverse two branches out of the node simultaneously and all branches are accounted for.

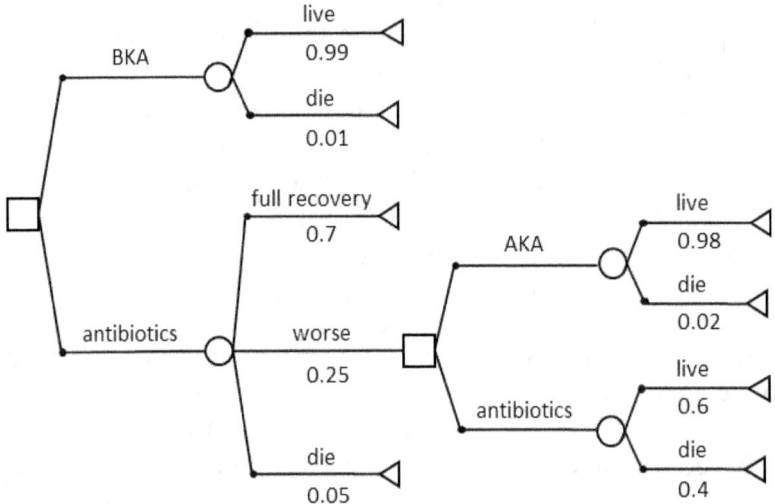

Figure 11-4 *Hypothetical decision tree faced by a patient who presents a gangrenous foot.*

A decision tree can have arbitrary branch structure. How branchy the tree is and how many nodes are in each root-to-leaf path is a modeling decision that would typically be made by the medical community or doctor. The goal of a decision tree is to help the patient understand treatment options, understand the potential outcomes from treatment, and help the patient ask the right questions to identify the right treatment. Branches from an action node should only correspond to actions that are considered reasonable, and not contraindicated by present medical understanding. In some cases, there may be branches from the root that correspond to "do nothing", watchful waiting, or active surveillance, among other treatment approaches.

Most medical decision trees that we find online have a branch structure that, except for the root, involves only chance nodes and leaves. This is not reflective of the fact that trees with subsequent decision nodes arise commonly in practice.

In Figure 11-4, the numbers under the branches are hypothetical probability estimates that would be obtained from historical data. Notice that for each node in the tree, the probabilities on the outgoing branches sum to one – reflecting the constraint that outgoing branches be exclusive and exhaustive. Seeing the branch probabilities is helpful to patients, but they're not always available. And even when they are, they're not always reliable, as would be the case if they were based on small samples The lack of reliable probability estimates in a decision tree is a clear signal that more data needs to be collected.

In general, a tree's branch structure and branch probabilities may change in time as more patient data comes in and new treatment technologies arrive.

Faced with a decision tree like that in Figure 11-4, the patient wants to answer the question: What is the best action to take at the root? The tree indicates four possible outcomes from treatment: full recovery; BKA; AKA; and death. In practice, the estimated probabilities in the tree would be based on a sample of historical patients. Within the subsample who followed the BKA branch out of the root, we can tally the four outcomes and create a probability histogram. The four bar probabilities are: full recovery (0); AKA (0); BKA (0.99); and death (0.1). Similarly, within the subsample of patients who followed the antibiotics branch out of the root, we can tally the four outcomes and create another probability histogram. In this case, the BKA bar has probability 0 while the other three bars all have non-zero probability. The current patient, trying to decide which action to take at the root, can compare these two histograms to assist in the decision.

(For the reader familiar with the concept of *folding back* a decision tree, the histograms for the actions at the root are equivalently obtained by a "modified" fold back that starts from the leaves and computes a probability-weighted "average of histograms" at both action nodes and chance nodes.)

Hip implant surgery

For any condition, a decision tree showing the various treatment options and potential paths forward can be useful in helping the patient ask the right questions and select the right treatment. What is the estimated probability of going down this chance branch? What is the corresponding confidence interval? What is the estimated success rate of this action branch? What is the probability distribution of performance on this action branch? Unfortunately, in many cases, only limited historical patient data is available for analysis. So the estimates we seek either don't exist or aren't very reliable. We see this, for example, when considering the different options available for hip implant surgery. We see it when considering surgical treatments for many other conditions as well. A decision tree can point to questions that are in need of more data, and make clear which treatments are more evidence-based than others. Patients can make better treatment decisions when they understand what is and what isn't known reliably.

Hip implant surgery is the most common orthopedic surgery in the world. It is performed on more than 300,000 patients a year in the US alone. Most often, hip implant surgery is undertaken to relieve chronic and painful osteoarthritis and restore mobility. (Taken together with knee replacements, the total number of patients receiving surgery in the US each year is over a million, according to a 2014 study by Mayo Clinic.)

There are two basic types of prosthesis available: total hip replacement (THR) and hip resurfacing arthroplasty (HRA). In total hip replacement (THR): the damaged femoral head is removed and then replaced with a long metal stem inserted into the femur and topped by a "small" metal (cobalt-chromium) or ceramic ball; the damaged bone and cartilage of the acetabulum is replaced with a metal socket; and a metal, ceramic, or plastic (polyethylene or cross-linked polyethylene) liner is inserted between the ball and socket to create a smooth gliding surface. Various ball-liner combinations are possible: Metal-on-Metal (MoM), Metal-on-Polyethylene (MoP), Ceramic-on-Metal (CoM), and others. There are several different installation approaches, and a variety of prosthetic designs to choose from.

Hip resurfacing (HRA) is a more bone-conserving approach: The femoral head is not removed, but instead trimmed and capped with a "large" metal shell. The damaged bone and cartilage of the acetabulum are again replaced with a metal socket. There is no liner. To our knowledge, Metal-on-Metal (MoM) is the only hip resurfacing option generally available today, while research with other materials continues. There is typically just one installation approach (posterior), and a variety of prosthetic designs to choose from. Hip resurfacing installation is more technically demanding than total hip replacement.

Either type of device can fail. Implant longevity may depend on various patient factors, such as gender, age, build, activity level, and bone quality. It may depend on the make and model of the device. When failure occurs, revision surgery is usually necessary. Reasons for implant failure include prosthetic loosening, implant wear and tear, particle and ion debris, femoral break (HRA), and repeated dislocation. If an HRA failure involves only the acetabular component, then there is the option of replacing just that component. If an HRA failure involves the femoral component, then the joint is typically converted to a THR (possibly with "large" femoral ball, if the original acetabular component is preserved). When converting from HRA to THR, the latter may have a shorter lifespan than a primary THR. (See "What is the re-revision rate after revising a hip resurfacing arthroplasty?", *Clin Orthop Relat Res.*, Nov. 2015.)

Studies of patients who received an HRA in the last ten to fifteen years suggest that certain models of the device have good-midterm performance, on par with THR, for the right kind of patient – the male patient under sixty with a robust-frame. Long-term data on HRA performance is not yet available. Proponent surgeons for HRA claim that, compared to THR, hip resurfacing provides better kinematic behavior in support of an active lifestyle, is less prone to dislocation, and offers greater implant longevity. At present, there seems to be little if any evidence backing up these claims:

From the Hip Resurfacing web page (last reviewed 2014) of the American Academy of Orthopedic Surgeons: *The advantages of hip resurfacing over traditional total hip replacements is an area of controversy among orthopedic surgeons. A great deal of research is currently being done on this topic.*

From the Hip Resurfacing web page (last updated 2016) on Medscape: *The clinical efficacy and cost-effectiveness of hip resurfacing in the long term have yet to be determined...No study has shown hip resurfacing to be superior to modern total hip replacements with regard to durability and survivorship.*

Figure 11-5 shows a decision tree for a 55-year old male who is seeking surgical treatment for an arthritic hip. The main decision is whether to go with hip resurfacing or total hip replacement. A key consideration is the number of anticipated revisions in the patient's lifetime, and trying to keep that number as low as possible.

A tree like that in Figure 11-5 shows the patient not only what might be in store, but also helps the patient ask the right questions to make the best treatment decision: What is the probability distribution of time-to-fail with this kind of device? In what sense is this device better than that device?

Other questions can be asked: Does the device shed harmful particles or ions? What percentage of patients are negatively affected? For THR, is it better to get anterior installation or posterior installation?

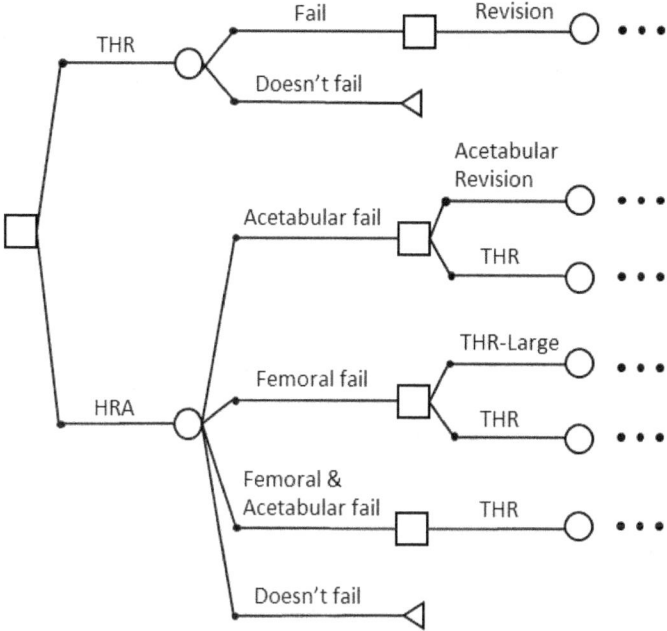

Figure 11-5 *A decision tree for a 55-year-old male patient who is considering surgical treatment for an arthritic hip. Ellipsis denotes continuation of the tree.*

Presently, with hip implant surgery, it's hard to get reliable, actionable answers to such questions. Many implant designs have only been around for a short time – so data on long-term performance (safety and efficacy) is scant or non-existent. New designs are not generally required to undergo clinical trials. Data on post-market device performance is slow to make its way to journal publications, and often the studies are only able to report on small sample sizes relative to specific questions of interest. The FDA is slow to issue warnings to doctors and the public. And various corrupting influences make it even more difficult for a patient to get reliable answers.

In fact, a lot of bad devices are out there in circulation. According to a 2013 *Consumer Union* report, "A Summary of Hip Implant Recalls", there were 578 recalls of hip implants and implant components between 2002 and 2013 by just six companies. Some of these companies are facing lawsuits from thousands of patients who claim to have been harmed by their implants. In 2016, Johnson & Johnson (DePuy Orthopedics) was ordered to pay out more than $1 billion on its metal-on-metal Pinnacle hip implants. In 2013, it paid out $2.5 billion on its ASR metal-on-metal implants. In these lawsuits, it is alleged that J&J (DePuy) did not warn consumers in a timely manner about elevated risks that were evident with these devices.

To our knowledge, most if not all of the problem hip implants mentioned above were cleared by the FDA through the 510(k) process, which does not require clinical trials to assess safety and efficacy, but instead considers manufacturer's arguments for "substantial equivalence" to predicate devices already on the market. (We mentioned the 510(k) process before in Chapter 4 in the section "Regulation of surgery and devices".) And since there are no animal models for testing these devices, it's the consumers who are the unwitting guinea pigs in tests of theory, and who frequently suffer the consequences.

When a device is put on the market, the manufacturer is required under US law to continue monitoring it for safety and efficacy, and to inform the public as soon as possible if problems occur and issue a recall. At the same time, the FDA gathers its own data and may recommend that a company launch a recall. Manufacturers are expected to issue recalls voluntarily, but far too often, companies drag their feet in a calculus that prioritizes sales over patient well-being. Furthermore, the FDA itself, being largely funded by user fees from the industries it regulates, cannot generally be relied upon to make a timely determination of when a product should be recalled. Upon seeing an initial set of studies that looks unfavorable, the agency often simply asks for more studies before showing any willingness to take action.

Eventually, studies get published in peer-reviewed medical journals. However, we find that trying to get actionable information from these articles is very difficult, if not impossible. Many studies cite numerous other studies. Studies do not always agree in their findings. There are many parameters to consider – and by the time you control for gender, age, activity level, build, bone quality, implant design, reason for revision, and so on, sample sizes are often too small to give reliable results for the current patient. (Limited patient data archives from the UK and Australia joint registries, both established in 2002, form the basis of many hip implant studies. Surprisingly, the US did not set up its own joint registry until 2012.) It's also unsettling how many authors of journal papers on devices acknowledge financial relationships with device manufacturers.

Patients cannot put blind faith in doctors to recommend the best type of implant. Dr. Chris Centeno writes in his online blog (last updated Dec. 2015): *Is your surgeon being paid to promote a certain type of hip? One of the real challenges [is that] joint replacement devices have been one of the worst areas of payola in medicine....many surgeons have figured out that they can keep their cash flow stable by taking money from the device manufacturers.*

It's all evidence of a grand collusion among device manufacturers, the FDA, lawmakers, and doctors pimping for the industry. It's a morass, and we, the patients, are caught up in it. Clearly, there's a desperate need for reliable data and standards, and for oversight to protect the patient from harms that he might have to cope with for the rest of his life.

We have focused on hip implant surgery, but collusion, corruption and payola are issues in many other areas of surgery. Knee and shoulder problems are often addressed surgically with the same lack of oversight and same lack of standards. Surgeries of the neck, back, hands and feet are often only weakly supported by statistical evidence. Claims made for ablation and pacemaker insertion to treat arrhythmia are often exaggerated well beyond their scientific support. In general, the problems of weak oversight and weak justification are rife in many kinds of surgery and are in desperate need of attention. The cost in dollars and health care quality is as incalculable as it is unacceptable.

Patients need to know if there is rigorous evidential basis for suggesting that surgery is the best way to go, and if so, which surgery and which device. They need to know if there are solid, reliable statistics to recommend one device over another, or if the "advantages" of a device are theoretical, or if a device is being promoted for some other reason. Patients need to understand if they are being used as guinea pigs. They need answers now – estimates, confidence intervals, histograms – based on the most extensive data available. They don't have time to wait around for journal articles to appear and professional consensus that may never come.

Leaning on the decision tree

When you come to a fork in the road, take it.

Yogi Berra

More than at any other time in history, mankind faces a crossroads. One path leads to despair and utter hopelessness; the other to total extinction. Let us pray we have the wisdom to choose correctly.

From "My Speech to the Graduates" by Woody Allen

We've seen a couple decision trees so far – we'll see some others in a moment. Again, the purpose of a decision tree is to help the patient understand the available treatment options, understand the potential outcomes from treatment, and help the patient ask the right questions to identify the right treatment. But, for the tree to be of greatest use, its branches should be outfitted with the relevant probabilities, confidence intervals, and probability distributions based on samples of historical patients who are similar to the current patient. That would reflect true personalized, evidence-based medicine.

The Angelina Jolie story

In 2013, famed Hollywood actress Angelina Jolie announced to the world that she had undergone preventative double mastectomy and would soon undergo preventative oophorectomy (removal of ovaries and fallopian tubes) as well, although she was only 37 years of age. Jolie carries a deleterious mutation of the *BRCA1* gene. Her mother had the gene mutation and died of ovarian cancer at age 56. (Jolie's mother died in 2007 after an eight-year battle with the disease). Given her genetics and family history, and the historical patient data at the time, Jolie's doctor concluded that her risk for breast cancer was 87% and for ovarian cancer was 50%. Treatment for either cancer had a very low success rate when linked to a deleterious *BRCA1* mutation. With prophylactic surgery, Jolie's doctor estimated her future cancer risk to be just 5% – well below the typical 12% lifetime risk for breast cancer. Figure 11-6 shows a decision tree like the one faced by Ms. Jolie.

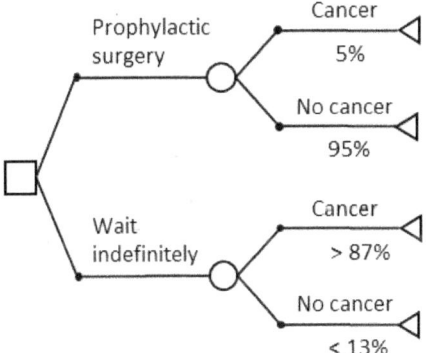

Figure 11-6 *A decision tree like the one faced by Angelina Jolie, given her BRCA1 gene mutation and family history.*

Up to 2013, medical experience indicated that breast and ovarian cancers, in the presence of a harmful *BRCA1* mutation, were very aggressive, and death due to such cancer was highly likely under any form of treatment.

In the article, "The Angelina Effect", *Time*, May 27, 2013, on page 33, we find some startling figures as to the approximate percentage of *BRCA1*-mutation-positive women who opt for preventative double mastectomy: 36% in the US; 0% in the Institute Curie in Paris; 100% in Northern Europe!

Such degree of variation is perplexing. The article speculates that it may be mostly due to social and cultural factors that influence personal tolerance for risk and uncertainty. We wonder if it has to do with availability of treatment. But it may also be fair to ask if it's due to ignorance among doctors and patients, or poor communication, regarding the cure rate of such cancers? That would heap extra tragedy on an already tragic situation.

Jolie's *BRCA1* mutation was there before birth. Her mother's diagnosis occurred when Jolie was 24 years old. This raises the question: If prophylactic surgery is the decided course of action, is age 37 the most prudent age at which to have the surgery?

In order to decide the "right" age at which to undergo prophylactic surgery, a patient would benefit from a fitted risk curve built from historical patient data. The curve would show, for each year of life X, the probability of being diagnosed with breast or ovarian cancer prior to age X, assuming no prophylactic surgery is performed. A confidence envelope could be displayed with this curve to indicate how reliable it is. If the risk curve shows a steep increase in the early forties, and a gradual slope prior, then that might point to the mid-thirties as the optimal time to have the surgery.

The Angelina Jolie story (continued)

When we first heard of Ms. Jolie's decision to have preemptive surgery, we were under the impression that breast or ovarian cancer in the presence of a deleterious *BRCA1* mutation was essentially a death sentence. This is not the case today, and there has been steady progress in extending the lives of those afflicted. Figure 11-7 shows a decision tree that Jolie might face today if she were deciding whether to pursue prophylactic surgery.

In Figure 11-7 we don't know the probabilities associated with the rightmost two chance branches, but estimates of those numbers and their confidence intervals would be highly useful for a patient's decision-making.

A similar decision tree comes into play for women who don't have deleterious *BRCA1* (or *BRCA2*) mutations but are diagnosed with ductal carcinoma in situ (DCIS), also called Stage 0 breast cancer, which accounts for about a quarter of breast cancers diagnosed in routine screening. As discussed in the article, "Why doctors are rethinking breast cancer treatment", *Time*, Oct. 12, 2015, DCIS, like prostate cancer, is often symptom-free and non-lethal. In this case, the question is: Should aggressive treatment be pursued – surgery, radiation, and chemotherapy, plus future surgical revisions – or a more conservative approach like watchful waiting or active surveillance? In the past, doctors commonly recommended aggressive treatment. But with recent studies showing that aggressive treatment for DCIS does not reduce mortality compared to the conservative approach, medical thought is shifting. Once again, it's all about the data!

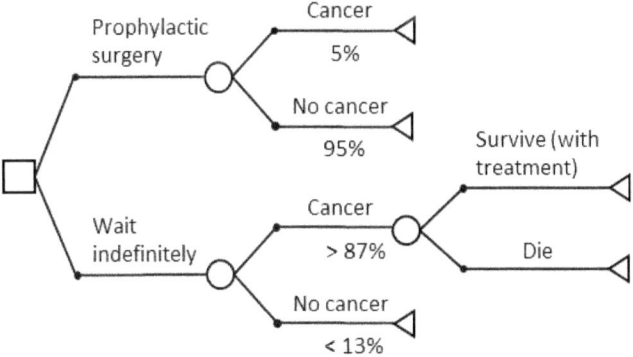

Figure 11-7 *A decision tree that Angelina Jolie might face today if she were contemplating prophylactic surgery.*

Aching back

X-rays and an MRI clinched the diagnosis – the pain in the butt, in the hip, and radiating down the leg of the 73-year old patient was due to a deteriorating disc between the lowermost lumbar vertebra L_5 and the uppermost sacral vertebra S_1. Lesser deterioration was observed in the discs between L_5 and L_4, and between L_4 and L_3. The surgeon laid-out two options: surgically stabilize L_5 to S_1, with the prospect that the other discs might need to be stabilized later (if patient age permits), or address L_3 to S_1 all at once. Figure 11-8 shows a decision tree corresponding to this situation.

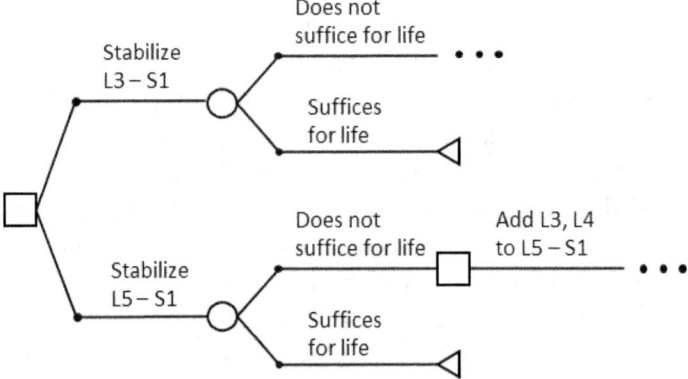

Figure 11-8 *A decision tree faced by a patient who needed back surgery to address disc deterioration in the spine. Ellipsis denote continuation of the tree.*

A phenomenon to bear mind with this kind of back surgery: the longer the stabilized section, the longer the recovery time, and the more rapid the deterioration of the discs adjacent to the stabilized section (the longer lever arm exerts more stress on the neighboring discs), a condition that might have to be addressed later.

What are the probabilities on the chance branches in the decision tree and what are their confidence intervals? Of course, we expect this to depend on patient age and perhaps other factors. What is the probability distribution on the length of time that stabilization surgery suffices?

When the patient asked the surgeon these kinds of questions, the surgeon said such statistics were not available! That doesn't pass as personalized, evidence-based medicine.

Prostate cancer

The lifetime risk for prostate cancer in the US is 14%, while the risk of dying from prostate cancer is 2.5%. (See "Lifetime Risk of Developing or Dying from Cancer" on the website cancer.org). Though prostate cancer is the second leading cause of cancer death among men in the US, in the great majority of cases it will be slow-growing and asymptomatic for life. In the great majority of men, aggressive treatment following the diagnosis of "prostate cancer" is over-treatment, exposing the patient to a high risk of harmful side effects while not extending life.

The most conservative approaches to addressing localized prostate cancer are watchful waiting and active surveillance. Aggressive treatments include radical prostatectomy, radiation therapy, cryotherapy, high-intensity focused ultra-sound, and focal laser ablation. Among aggressive treatments, there is no single approach that is considered universally best — each has its advantages and disadvantages. Aggressive treatments can lead to serious side effects such as impotence, incontinence, and rectal damage.

There was a time when the PSA screening test was considered a reliable indicator of aggressive prostate cancer. But in 2012, based on large studies, the US Preventative Services Task Force (USPSTF) concluded (quote): *the benefit of PSA screening does not outweigh the potential risks, which include pain, fever, bleeding, infection and problems urinating, resulting from biopsies as well as incontinence and impotence associated with the treatment of tumors that would not have otherwise caused harm. Each year, about [1200] men die from complications associated with treatments prompted by PSA screening.* The Task Force goes on to say that routine PSA screening and early treatment protects at most 1 in 1,000 men from death due to prostate cancer. The Task Force now recommends against routine PSA screening.

Figure 11-9 shows a pair of decision trees. One is for the diagnosis of prostate cancer, and begins with consideration of symptoms, family history, health history, and digital rectal exam (DRE). The other is for the treatment of localized prostate cancer. The patient is naturally concerned about length of life and quality of life.

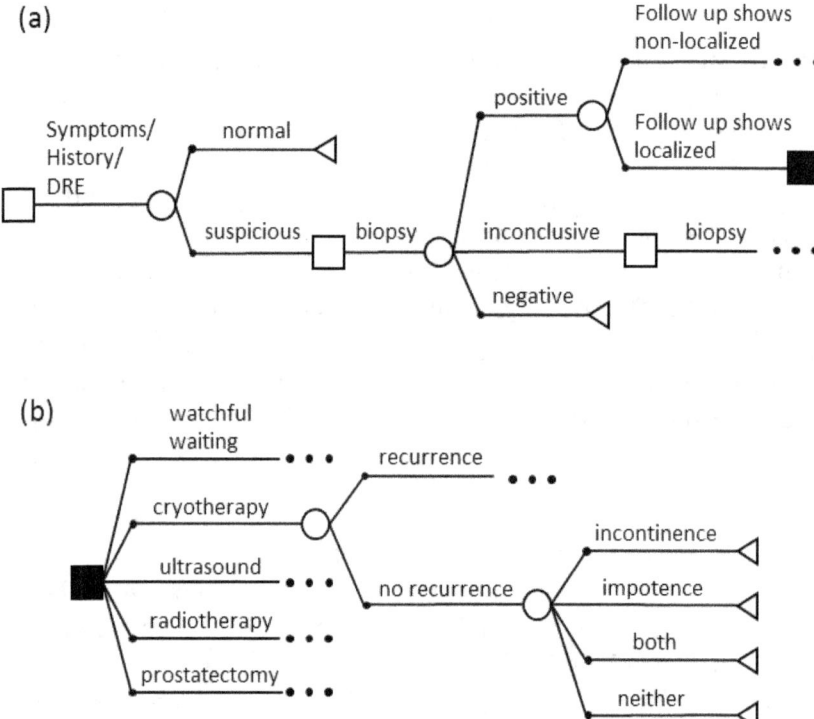

Figure 11-9 *(a) A decision tree for the diagnosis of prostate cancer; (b) A decision tree for the treatment of (localized) prostate cancer. Ellipsis denote continuation of the tree. The two black squares represent the same action node.*

The patient would benefit from answers to the following kinds of questions: What is the difference in mortality rate between, watchful waiting, active surveillance, and immediate aggressive treatment? What are those rates and what are their confidence intervals? For each aggressive treatment, what is the probability of recurrence and what are the confidence intervals? What is the probability that the treatment will lead to incontinence or impotence, or both, and what are the confidence intervals?

In a heartbeat

Atrial fibrillation, A-fib for short, is the most common, serious abnormal heart rhythm. A-fib and atrial flutter resulted in 112,000 deaths in 2013. It is most often a progressive condition and has a low cure rate. Treatment usually begins with a drug regimen and lifestyle changes, but later could involve a modified drug regimen and one or more invasive "rhythm control" procedures, such as pacemaker installation, ablation of heart tissue, or most extreme of all, complete disabling of the atrioventricular (AV) node (also necessitating pacemaker installation). Figure 11-10 shows the sort of decision tree that a patient may face when considering the various invasive procedures for A-fib. The patient is looking to limit the risks associated with treatment, while seeking to maintain a high quality of life (e.g., less fatigue).

The patient would benefit from answers to the following sorts of questions: What is the probability that moderate or persistent A-fib will return after ablation, and with what confidence intervals? What is the probability distribution of that recurrence time? The same questions can be asked for pacemaker installation. Unfortunately, to our understanding, these statistics are not yet available. From the NIH webpage (last updated Sept. 2014) for the National Heart, Lung, and Blood Institute, answering the question "How is Atrial Fibrillation Treated?", there is the quote: *The long-term benefits of rhythm control have not been proven conclusively yet... Research on the benefits of catheter ablation as a treatment for AF is still ongoing.*

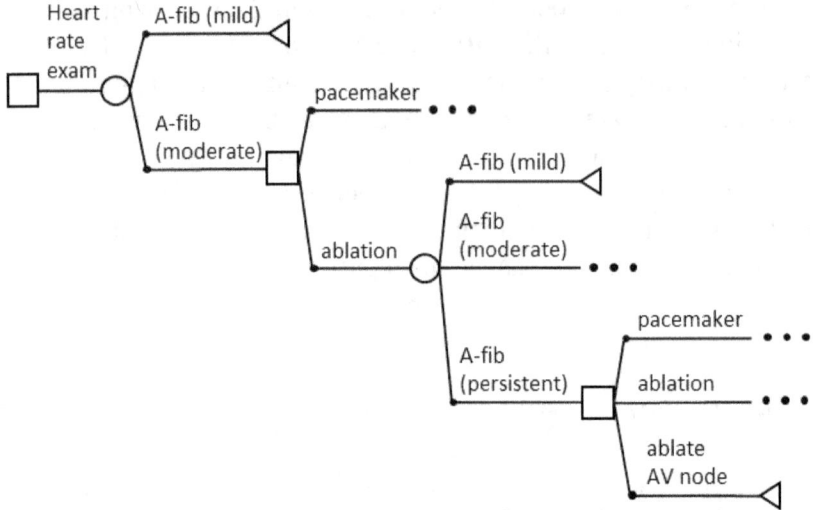

Figure 11-10 *The sort of decision tree that a patient might face when considering invasive treatments for atrial fibrillation. Ellipsis denote continuation of the tree.*

The Rolling Stones put it this way...

You can't always get what you want. But if you try sometimes, you just might find, you get what you need.

Regrettably it's true – you can't always get what you want. And sometimes, even when you try, you might not be able to get what you need. You may want a drug to cure a certain condition, or an operation that will correct a certain infirmity. But such a drug or procedure might not yet exist. That said, in vastly many other instances, medical technology, though it may come up short in getting you what you want, is often able to give you what you need – be it sufficient relief from discomfort so that you can maintain a certain quality of life, or peace of mind that comes from reducing the risk of a catastrophic health event.

You may want to know with certainty the success rate of a treatment, but since the relevant population may be very large or largely inaccessible, you may have to settle for a statistical estimate and confidence interval based on an unbiased sample of historical patients. But that is often sufficient for enabling you to make a reasoned decision about which treatment to go with. So you get what you need.

Part III

Towards Rigorous, Personalized, Evidence-Based Medicine

Ch. 12: *79.48% of statistics are made up on the spot*

attribution????

If personalized, evidence-based medicine is what you want, then rigorous statistics on historical patient data is your best guide. Yet, many disagree. They view all statistics as unreliable and untrustworthy. They see numbers tossed about to persuade and sell stuff – products, services, points of view – sometimes even nefarious stuff. They see numbers whose origins are not explained and that lack any guarantee of reliability. They see pundits basing claims on these numbers – claims that often prove to be incorrect.

Some people call these numbers "statistics" – we call them flimflam stats. These numbers should not be confused with numbers arrived at through the framework we've been discussing. The latter numbers can be rightly called rigorous statistics, because they do come with a guarantee of reliability, a guarantee that is universally understood and accepted. This kind of statistics you ignore at your peril.

"Statistics" leading us astray

If you want to make someone believe in something that is really, really stupid, just stick a number on it.

Charles Seife

Rigorous statistics refers to a methodology for collecting and analyzing samples in order to reach provisional conclusions about a population, conclusions accompanied by objective measures of reliability given as confidence intervals. The methodology is based on the incontrovertible mathematics of chapters 7 - 10. The methodology requires that samples be unbiased, and that sample-based conclusions be consistent with sample size. In a rigorous statistical study, there is full disclosure regarding sample selection, measurement, and analysis, and of course, honest reporting of results. Full disclosure allows for meaningful review and scrutiny by others. A conscientious reviewer will reject a study for publication if there is good reason to believe that the study sample or measurement technique is biased.

In a rigorous statistical study, if the measurement of interest is on a continuous scale (e.g., body height, IQ, longevity), and if the sample mean is offered as an estimate of the population mean, then additionally, the sample standard deviation is offered as an estimate of the population standard deviation together with a confidence interval. Whether estimating a population mean, standard deviation, histogram, bar chart, curve fit, or anything else, a rigorous statistical study always characterizes the reliability of its results.

A rigorous statistical study is *reproducible* to the degree indicated by the confidence interval. Assuming the population mean lies within, say, the 95% confidence interval of the sample mean, and new studies (of the same size as the first study) are run, then 95% of these new sample means will be no further from the first sample mean than the width of the confidence interval.

Numbers not obtained using rigorous statistical methodology fall into the realm of **flimflam stats** ("flimflam" meaning "deceptive" or "nonsensical") and should be regarded with skepticism. Flimflam stats are frequently unreliable. Though sometimes their purpose is well-intentioned, often they are used to bamboozle. Flimflam stats come in a variety of flavors including: claims without meaningful confidence measures, claims based on biased samples, claims based on anecdote, claims based on non-rigorous meta-studies, extrapolation based on controversial assumptions, cherry-picking of results, cover-ups, and cooking the books. Here are some examples:

- *The sky is falling!* So cried Chicken Little centuries ago. The warning was echoed by Reverend Thomas Malthus in 1798: Exponential population growth will overwhelm the resources needed to support it.

  The banner was taken up again in 1972 with the publication of the book *The Limits of Growth* by a team of researchers at MIT, funded by The Club of Rome. The book was laden with data, computer models and apocalyptic forecasts: In thirty years, we will run short of fossil fuels, arable lands, and ocean bounties. Clearly, the predictions did not pan out.

  Then, in 2001, Bjorn Lomborg, adjunct professor at the Copenhagen Business School, presented an entirely different view in his book *The Skeptical Environmentalist*. There he maintained that predictions of overpopulation, declining energy resources, water and food shortages, pollution, and other such disasters were unsupported, and he offered copious data to back up his claims. The book ignited a firestorm of protests from legions of environmental scientists who accused Lomborg of scientific dishonesty and deliberately presenting misleading data. Is Lomborg leading us astray? The debate continues.

- The earth is cooling, the new ice age cometh – that was the mantra of the 1960's. It's what the science showed then, according to the overwhelming majority of climatologists – and they had the data to back it up.

- Remember the hoopla in support of the hydrogen economy? Proponents had the numbers to back the approach. But now the idea appears to have run out of gas. Evidently, the total cost of obtaining, shipping, and storing the hydrogen was not as well-understood as initially thought.

- Then there was the push for biofuels. Some promoted the fermenting of sea weed and water hyacinth. Others pushed for extracting combustibles from corn – perfectly good corn that could be used for fodder or whisky mash. All of these schemes came complete with supporting data. But critics argue that the biofuel approach is not competitive with conventional energy sources.

- For decades, recommendations based on studies have flip-flopped on whether a particular food, food component, or beverage is bad for you, good for you, or neutral. These include eggs, salt, saturated fat, carbohydrates, shrimp, beef, and wine.

- Politicians and political scientists always manage to find cadres of statisticians who identify themselves with the right, or the left, or the center, and are seldom at a loss to find numbers that support their views on taxation, regulation, minimum wage, energy, trade, healthcare, and so on.

- Economists, too, seldom hold forth without some attempt to find statistical cover for their nakedness. Again, there are right-leaning, left-leaning, and center-leaning economists, Keynesians, and followers of Adam Smith. Whatever their inclination, they are rarely at a loss to find numbers to support their views, or the views they are paid to support.

- Drawing conclusions from anecdote is another way we can be led astray. While American novelist Mark Twain was in London in 1897, rumor spread that he had fallen gravely ill. Then rumor spread that he had died. Later, Twain famously quipped: *The reports of my death have been greatly exaggerated.* (The quip is actually due to Twain biographer Albert Paine. Twain's true response was uncharacteristically less inspired.)

- Big Pharma and medical device manufacturers, are not above bending or cherry-picking the numbers to suite their purposes. And those purposes are not always to best serve patients, doctors, and healthcare, but to sell stuff – with claims of improving health, comfort, libido, and appearance, in order to promote a younger, stronger, sexier you.

- Violence has been declining over the course of history – so says Steven Pinker, professor of psychology at Harvard. In his book, *The Better Angels of our Nature*: *Why Violence has Declined* (2011), he goes back to the Middle Ages, to the days of knights and nobility to argue his point, neglecting many centuries and many cultures through time, some so peaceful that they didn't even have a word for war. Today, the population in the Mid-East alone is greater than the world's population in medieval times, and we rather doubt they would accept Pinker's premise.

- Disparity of individual wealth in the US is exploding according to some interpretations of the data; not so according to others. If you're comparing the 1970's with the last 25 years, the exploding disparity is clear; if you're comparing the 1920's and 30's with the last 25 years, wealth inequality in the US is about the same. Which narrative you choose has huge social and political implications. (Google "wealth inequality is now as bad as in the 1920s".)

- Big Tobacco publicly denied the causal link between cigarette smoking and cancer until 1994, even though their own internal studies, going as far back as the 1950's, indicated otherwise. They also denied that nicotine is addictive and that secondhand smoke is harmful – again contradicting their own studies.

Similar deceit was perpetrated by the asbestos industry, which denied the causal link between asbestos inhalation and cancer.

- *Wall Street Week* was a PBS weekly television show hosted by Louis Rukeyser that ran from 1970 to 2002 and discussed financial news and financial markets. The show regularly featured ten technical analysts, dubbed the "elves" by Rukeyser, who attempted to predict the direction of the market in the following months. They gained popularity from their consistent inability to make correct predictions.

- For years the NFL dismissed the link between playing football and traumatic brain injury. They even commissioned their own research studies, which used cherry-picked data to argue that NFL players were quick to recover from concussions.

- "Dewey Defeats Truman" read the headline of the *Chicago Daily Tribune* the morning after the 1948 US presidential election, prompting Truman to retort, "That ain't the way I heard it," after his upset victory over Dewey. Three major polling agencies, including Gallup, predicted Dewey would win. How did things go awry? A mix of stopping the polling too soon and failing to guard against sample bias. Concerning the latter: Much of the polling was done by telephone. The telephone was a luxury at that time, limited to more prosperous households, and Truman was less popular among that class of voters.

  In the 2016 US presidential election, virtually every major polling agency predicted that Clinton would defeat Trump. What went wrong?

Here's another example of flimflam stats, one that represents an abuse of math, statistics, and computer science, all at once. The offending parties are Lu Hong, professor of business at Loyola University Chicago, and Scott Page, professor of political science at the University of Michigan. Their paper, "Groups of diverse problem solvers can outperform groups of high-ability problem solvers", first appeared in the prestigious Proceedings of the National Academy of Sciences in 2004, and then was further elaborated on in Page's book, *The Difference*, in 2007. The claim is that diversity trumps ability, that a diverse group of non-exceptional individuals is better at problem-solving than a talented group of like-minded experts. Page states in his book: *...the veracity of the diversity trumps ability claim is not a matter of dispute. It's true, just as 1+1 = 2 is true.*

However, Abigail Thompson, professor of mathematics at the University of California, Davis, begs to differ. In her article, "Does diversity trump ability? An example of the misuse of statistics in the social sciences", *Notices of the American Mathematics Society*, Oct. 2014, she debunks the research top-to-bottom, arguing that math it isn't; statistics it isn't; computer science it isn't; and that the pertinence of their research to the thesis under discussion is far-fetched at best. *Just as true as 1+1=2 is true...*what nonsense!

But the work by Lu Hong and Scott Page gained considerable traction and has been widely cited. We wonder what has been its effect on academia and industry.

Before we leave this example, there's an additional point we'd like to make: In the opening paragraphs of Dr. Thompson's paper, she admonishes the mathematics community for showing little interest in debunking works in other fields that use math and statistics to give their work the appearance of rigor, when in fact there is no rigor. Unfortunately, Dr. Thompson's paper, for all its merits, is not the kind of article that gets the math community fired up, or that gets credit as a valuable service at many colleges and universities. Such efforts are under-appreciated by math departments and do little to advance the career of an academic mathematician. Too bad. Such papers should be considered valuable contributions to the scientific community and to the public served by science.

So how to incentivize mathematically-trained academics to write such papers? What about setting up departments dedicated to mathematical review of journal publications in other fields, especially publications that are highly cited? This would serve to keep standards high in those fields.

Many of the examples above came from media headlines, but only a few of them are of direct medical interest. But there are plenty of examples of flimflam stats in medicine:

- The great majority of implantable devices are not cleared for market on the basis of FDA clinical trials, but rather through the FDA's 510(k) process where the manufacturer need only argue substantial design equivalence to a previously cleared "predicate" device. Claiming efficacy and safety for a new device based on performance data for a predicate is a claim based on flimflam stats.

- FDA clinical trials for new drugs are usually only about five years long in total. Claiming long term efficacy and safety based on short term efficacy and safety is a claim based on flimflam stats.

- Promoting a new surgical procedure without rigorous statistics on efficacy and safety is a recommendation based on flimflam stats.

- Off-label drug prescription without rigorous statistics on efficacy and safety is a prescription based on flimflam stats.

- In the realm of pre-clinical, biomedical research, many research results in scientific journals are not reproducible. (See, for example, the article, "1500 scientists lift the lid on reproducibility", *Nature*, May 25, 2016.)

- In 1998, Dr. Andrew Wakefield and a team of colleagues published an article in *The Lancet*, based on a study of 12 autistic children, in which they proposed a link between autism and the measles-mumps-rubella (MMR) triple vaccine. Shortly after, Wakefield held a press conference and called for suspension of the MMR vaccine until more research could be done. He recommended individual vaccinations for the three diseases, separated by one year. (A 2005 study done in Japan, where separate vaccinations had been used since 1993, showed no difference in autism rates between those who received single shots and those who received the MMR shot.)

Subsequently, MMR vaccination rates in the US, Canada, UK and Europe, began to fall as parents became concerned about the risk of autism after vaccination. This led to a corresponding rise in measles and mumps, in some cases resulting in serious illness and death. Wakefield's continued warnings against the MMR vaccine have created a climate of distrust about all vaccines, causing the re-emergence of other previously controlled diseases.

Following Wakefield's 1998 paper, other studies were published – none able to confirm a correlation between MMR vaccination and autism. Wakefield has refused to repeat his study using a larger more randomized sample. In 2004, ten out of the twelve coauthors on the paper issued a retraction in the *The Lancet*, stating that "no causal link was established between MMR vaccine and autism, as the data were insufficient". In 2010, *The Lancet* itself retracted the paper, criticizing the authors for selective sampling, fraudulent reporting of results, and non-disclosure of financial conflicts of interests (e.g., Wakefield received funding from lawyers representing parents of children in the study who were bringing suit against vaccine manufacturers.) If you look online for the 1998 Wakefield paper in *The Lancet*, you will see it plastered with big red letters: "RETRACTED". (See Wikipedia, "Andrew Wakefield".)

- Lyme disease affects roughly 300,000 people a year in the US, and 65,000 people a year in Europe. In 1998, a vaccine for Lyme disease, called LYMErix, was approved by the FDA. In clinical trials with more than 10,000 people, the vaccine effectiveness was observed to be 76% among adults and 100% among children, with only mild or moderate transient adverse effects. Post-market, however, hundreds of consumers reported they had developed autoimmune side effects from the vaccine, and filed class-action lawsuits against the manufacturer. Curiously, when both the FDA and CDC investigated, they found no correlation. Eventually, negative media coverage caused sales of the vaccine to plummet, and in 2002 the manufacturer pulled the vaccine off the market. Today, there is still no Lyme vaccine for humans, but there is for your dog. We wonder: Were flimflam stats at play in this episode? Was LYMErix rightly taken off the market?

Rigorous statistics are the antidote to flimflam stats.

The medium is the message

Marshall McLuhan

That's how McLuhan put it, referring to the way in which the platform influences the perception of the message coming from it. In particular, TV, radio, lecterns, and pulpits are an integral part of any message delivered from them, shaping its meaning, impact, and credibility.

An oration soapboxed from a makeshift podium on a tidy lawn won't be taken as seriously as one broadcast from the Oval Office. George W. Bush's 2003 televised speech from the deck of an aircraft carrier proclaiming "mission accomplished" (in Iraq) would not have been nearly as impressive had it been delivered from a pier on Coney Island. John F. Kennedy's 1962 televised evening speech on the Cuban Missile Crisis would not have been nearly as impactful had it first been posted in the morning papers. So, depending on the medium, the message originating from it may have more or less gravity, more or less credibility, or more or less humor.

In the medical realm, there is no more impressive medium than a high-tech, medical instrument. Take for example, a thermographic imaging machine. It creates remarkable, colorized, infrared images showing the patterns of heat and blood flow on or near the surface of the body. Thermographic devices have been cleared by the FDA for use as an adjunct tool with traditional 2D X-ray mammography for detecting breast cancer. But for a number of years, various health care providers were claiming that thermal imaging can take the place of traditional mammography; that it can detect breast cancer years before detection by mammogram. No rigorous statistical studies support this claim and in 2011 the FDA began sending cease and desist letters to those promoting it, like quackster-in-chief, Dr. Joseph Mercola. (See "Thermogram No Substitute for Mammogram" at fda.gov).

A brand can be a medium. Dr. Scholl's, the well-recognized foot care company, has a long history of providing reputable products like cushion and gel insoles, and special pads to deal with warts, calluses, and corns. These days they also sell a line of "magnetic energy" insoles that deliver "revolutionary magnetic therapy". Being a product from the well-respected Dr. Scholl's, these insoles must be very effective – except that there is no rigorous evidence to suggest that they're any better than the cheaper models without magnetic energy.

Even the doctor's office is a medium. The generous desk, the book-lined shelves, the assorted paraphernalia neatly and visibly displayed – all bound to impress the patient with an aura of experience, expertise, and knowledge-based judgement.

A medium can be a fancy piece of software accessed by smart pad or desktop computer. Take, for example, diagnostic decision support (DDX) systems. A representative is Isabel, by Isabel Healthcare. (Others include DXplain and VisualIDx). Given the patient's symptoms and EMR, it provides a ranked list of diagnoses for the doctor to consider.

According to a company whitepaper last updated in 2016, Isabel uses (quote): *statistical natural language processing applied to a database of over 10,000 diagnosis presentations or illness scripts*. Sounds impressive. To its credit, the whitepaper gives links to recent studies and objective reviews of DDX systems. One of the articles, "The Effectiveness of Electronic

Differential Diagnoses Generators: A Systematic Review and Meta-Analysis", *PloS One*, Mar. 8, 2016, states: *[Such] generators did not demonstrate improved diagnostic retrieval compared to clinicians. ... [They] have the potential to increase diagnostic uncertainty. Data on the number of investigations ordered and on cost-effectiveness remain inconclusive. ... [They] have the potential to improve diagnostic practice among clinicians. However, the high levels of heterogeneity, the variable quality of the reported data and the minimal benefits observed for complex cases suggest caution. Further research needs to be undertaken ... before their use in routine clinical practice can be recommended.*

Isabel is promoted to doctors and hospitals with claims that it leads to higher diagnostic accuracy, and that it enhances patient satisfaction: *[Seeing the doctor use a diagnostic decision support tool] has been shown to significantly increase satisfaction, as the patient feels as though they are being listened to and are reassured that a thorough assessment is being done.*

Patients and doctors see a snazzy, techy, computer interface, and are told a few buzzwords about what's under the hood, and many are immediately sold on its credibility and usefulness. They don't ask to see the rigorous statistics comparing machine performance with human performance. It's another example of what we need to be cautious about in medicine: taking the medium as the message. The medium may look credible and convincing, but the message may be useless or wrong.

The gravelly, stentorian voice of former US Secretary of State, Dr. Henry Kissinger, with its gravitas and authority, is itself a medium. Who dare challenge a voice like that?

Linus Pauling (1901 – 1994) won the Nobel prize for chemistry in 1954 for research into the nature of chemical bonds and insights into the structure of complex substances. Pauling eventually worked out the molecular structure of hemoglobin and explained the molecular cause of sickle-cell anemia. To this day, his fame and prestige make his views on almost anything widely influential. Unfortunately, toward the end of his career, he no longer adhered to the high standards of scientific rigor that he practiced earlier in his career.

In the 1970's, Pauling wrote three popular books extolling the virtues of mega-dose vitamin C, claiming that it reduces the duration and severity of both the common cold and flu, and that it is effective in fighting cancer. Rigorous statistical studies do not support any of these claims. Also during this period, Pauling helped lead the health-food industry's campaign to weaken the FDA's authority to protect consumers from misleading nutrition claims. (See quackwatch.com, "The dark side of Linus Pauling's legacy".) But with the never-ending mindset, "he's so smart he couldn't possibly be wrong" (to cite the title of a YouTube video on Pauling), annual sales of vitamin C have been sky-high for decades.

Sir Ronald Fisher (1890 – 1962), called by some "the father of modern statistics", spoke out against the 1950 study that strongly suggested a link between smoking and lung cancer – arguing that correlation does not imply causation. Fisher was unwilling to entertain such a link likely because of the personal solace he himself found in tobacco. (See Wikipedia, "Ronald Fisher".) Like Pauling, here was an intellectual giant with an awesome power to move minds – sometimes in the wrong direction.

Direct-to-consumer advertising of drugs through television, magazines, and the internet is another way we fall for "the medium is the message". These ads show inspiring images of life being lived to the fullest, but offer no rigorous statements on efficacy and safety, and no rigorous comparisons to other drugs. Yet, the ads are very successful in getting patients to pressure their doctors for a prescription. As pointed out earlier in the book, the US is one of only two countries in the world where direct-to-consumer adverting is even allowed – the other being New Zealand. Other countries recognize the danger of this practice to both patient and healthcare system: new drugs may be neither as safe nor as effective as existing drugs, while costing more.

In other advertisements, anti-oxidants are touted in food products, beverages, and supplements. Though anti-oxidants are all the rage, there is no rigorous statistical evidence suggesting that a boost in anti-oxidants promotes health, quality of life, or longevity. There are, however, a number of studies suggesting the opposite, that loading up on anti-oxidants somewhat reduces longevity. The Oxidation Theory of Aging (also called the Free Radical Theory of Aging) was originated by chemist Denham Harmon in the 1950's, and posits that cellular damage due to oxidation by free radicals is the key driver in aging. Today, studies show that oxidative damage is as much a byproduct of aging as a driver of aging, and that consuming large amounts of anti-oxidants is not only not beneficial, but may be deleterious. It appears that some amount of oxidation stimulates the *self-healing* ability of cells, which may actually extend life. (See "The Myth of Antioxidants", *Scientific American*, Jan. 2013.)

A similar advertising campaign exists for probiotic foods and drinks. Though rigorous statistical evidence suggests that probiotics are helpful to some people – namely those taking antibiotics, or who have irritable bowel syndrome, or are in neonatal intensive care – there is no such evidence indicating any benefit to healthy people. (See "Do Probiotics Really Work?", *Scientific American*, July 2017.)

Infomercials feature well-known TV personalities like Dr. Andrew Weil, Dr. Mark Hyman, Dr. David Perlmutter, and Dr. Daniel Amen, all promoting their medical philosophies on stage before live studio audiences. Dr. Mehmet Oz, another TV personality, has his own show. These people have advanced degrees and are masters of public presentation – projecting authority, knowledge, and experience. Because of that skill, they are widely viewed as experts by the public. Yet the "medicine" they espouse is not supported by rigorous statistical evidence and not worthy of your trust. Here's a quote from one of Dr. Hyman's infomercials: *The way we think about disease, mental illness, and our brain aging, actually has nothing to do with how our body actually works... The way we think about disease is all wrong... the name of the disease tells us nothing about the real reason or the causes of them. Diseases don't exist.*

Really? – Diseases don't exist?

Furthermore, Dr. Hyman, Dr. Oz, and Dr. Joseph Mercola, all Quackwatch notables, make unsubstantiated claims about the harms of vaccination, to the detriment of all of us.

Demanding rigorous statistics protects us from succumbing to "the medium is the message".

From casino to clinic

The incontrovertible mathematics covered in the previous five chapters is the bedrock of rigorous statistics, enabling sample-based estimates of a population to be accompanied by confidence intervals. It turns out, this same mathematics allows us to compute the odds of certain medical outcomes with *perfect* accuracy and confidence by leveraging the equivalence between biological mechanisms and casino games that involve fair coins and fair dice. For example, there is a well-validated connection between idealized coin tossing experiments and the inheritance patterns of certain genetic disorders such as cystic fibrosis, sickle-cell anemia, muscular dystrophy, Huntington disease, and Tay-Sachs disease. This connection enables genetic counselors to state, with perfect accuracy and confidence, the probability that a child of prospective parents will inherit such a disease. (For instance, if you Google "inheritance patterns for single-gene disorders", you'll see diagrams for autosomal dominant, autosomal recessive, X-linked dominant, and X-linked recessive diseases, all of whose inheritance patterns mirror the probabilistic outcomes of idealized coin tossing experiments.)

We saw this sort of connection in Example 7 in Chapter 7, when we were talking about coat color inheritance in Doberman pinschers. Here's an even simpler example:

Most of our genes are present in pairs, one member of the pair coming from our father and the other from our mother. The members of a pair can be identical or somewhat different. Let's focus on a gene pair whose members are different, and let's denote those members H and T.

When cell division creates a sex cell (an egg or sperm), only one member of the gene pair is allocated to the cell. So a given sex cell will contain exactly one of H or T, with 50-50 odds, just like tossing a fair coin with H being heads and T being tails. So uniting a sperm and an egg to create an embryo is like tossing two fair coins. The result is an embryo of type HH 25% of the time, type TT 25% of the time, and HT 50% of the time.

One member of the gene pair, say T, might be *recessive* and the other, say H, might be *dominant* – this in the sense that expression of the recessive member is masked by the dominant member. This is the case with many important diseases such as cystic fibrosis, sickle-cell anemia, and Tay-Sachs disease. In these cases, only the TT offspring will have the disease – HH offspring will not, and HT offspring will be *carriers* of the disease.

Suppose DNA analysis shows that the prospective parents are both carriers – that both are HT. The concern is that a child might be TT, the double dose assuring that the child will have the disease. Without equivocating, the genetic counselor can say that, on average, one out of four of their kids will have the disease, two out of four will be carriers like the parents, and one out of four will neither have the disease nor be a carrier.

The genetic counselor might have to explain that not every family with four kids will turn out that way – just *on average* will it turn out that way. In some families with two HT parents, there might be three that have the disease and one might be a carrier, or none might have the disease, and so on – all combinations are possible, and probability theory gives you the probability of each possibility – gives it to you unequivocally.

Of course, knowing the probabilities, even with perfect certainty, does not tell prospective parents what they should do – it simply informs them of the risk they're taking if they decide to conceive. The parent's decision to conceive or not conceive will depend on their personal values and possibly their views on prenatal testing and on terminating pregnancy if the fetus should have the disease.

Various multi-gene human traits also have inheritance patterns that are well-modeled by idealized coin-tossing experiments: skin color, hair color, eye color, and ABO blood type.

So again, we see the importance of mathematics in medical understanding and decision-making.

Why isn't rigorous statistics used more in medicine?

Demanding rigorous statistics avoids the hazards of flimflam stats and "the medium is the message". This is of particular importance in medicine, where too much treatment does not have rigorous evidential support. This serves neither the patient nor the healthcare system.

But a more rigorous approach to medicine is possible and has been for a while. It involves computerized, rigorous statistical analysis on standardized EMR's of historical patients who are like the current patient. So, why aren't we doing it? Why is it taking so long? Why, in these times, were EMR's not mandated until 2009? There are several answers:

Over the centuries, medicine was practiced through the patient-doctor interaction, where the doctor was sole decision-maker on diagnosis and treatment, the decisions based on personal experience, training, intuition, and rules of thumb. Patients have come to expect this kind of interaction.

This traditional way of thinking still strongly influences the way medicine is practiced today, the way medical information is reported in the media, and the way drug and device companies promote their products. How often do we hear the statement "Ask your doctor if this drug is right for you."

One reason for the attachment to the traditional paradigm is that many doctors lack understanding of basic statistical concepts. Many physicians do not understand what rigorous statistics is, nor why it is the best way to arrive at patient-centric, medical decisions.

Some physicians fear that computers offering rigorous advice on best-practice medical care will diminish their professional prestige, reduce the number of procedures they perform, subtract from the bottom line, and possibly put them out of a job.

In the June 27, 2015 issue of *The Washington Post*, the article "Watson's next feat? Taking on cancer – IBM's computer brain is training alongside doctors to do what they can't" says (quote): *But the Watson project and similar initiatives also have raised speculation – and alarm – that companies are seeking to replace the nation's approximately 900,000 physicians with software [...] Many physicians and academics in medicine have come to view Watson's work with reservation, despite reassurances from IBM officials that they are trying not to replace humans but to help them do their jobs better.*

From the Isabel Healthcare whitepaper mentioned in the previous section (quote): *With the excitement about computers and artificial intelligence (AI) of the 1960-1980's, many system developers [...] were too ambitious about what the computer could do. Trying to build systems that could mimic and then replace clinicians, led to a lack of general acceptance of the technology.*

Though in a curious double-think, the same whitepaper states: *The computer will never be able to tell the clinician what the patient's diagnosis is, as it never has all the contextual information about the patient...*

Patients don't ask their doctors for rigorous statistics on treatment partly because they don't understand what rigorous statistics means, and partly because patients are used to deferring to their doctor's judgement. Many patients are reluctant to accept that rigorous statistics applied to a population of strangers could possibly be relevant to their own specific situation. They may be skeptical that a computer analysis on abstract data points could possibly be more personalized than the judgement of the human doctor standing in front of them.

Legislators of public health policy often have little if any knowledge of basic statistical concepts. For them its often more about serving a lobby or political or personal agenda than doing what's best for patients and the healthcare system.

So where should you put your trust?

Looking for abuses of statistics? There are many examples all around us. But that shouldn't close our minds to the enormous benefits that *rigorous statistics* can bring to medical practice. Rigorous statistics will usher in far better health care at more affordable cost. The prerequisites are there and ready to go: the mathematical and statistical support; the computing power; and the data in the form of standardized EMR's. We can no longer afford to blindly follow the old school ways. It's far too costly, both in money and quality of health care. We now have the means to change and we shouldn't settle for less.

Ch. 13 Nothing but the Best

Isn't that what we all want, nothing by the best? Especially in health care, we want the best drugs, the best treatments, and the best outcomes. Unfortunately, in the US, what we often get is lousy health care at ruinous costs.

The per-capita cost of healthcare in the US is two to three times that of other major industrialized nations. In 2016, US healthcare expenditures were 17.8% of GDP, with an annual per-capita cost of $10,345. By 2025, it is predicted to be 20% of GDP. And what does this buy for us? Among other things, it buys us a lot of over-treatment, ineffective and harmful treatment, unnecessary medical tests, and large numbers of avoidable medical errors by doctors and hospitals. Much of this indicates a lack of standards and a failure by the medical community to adopt a modern approach to medical decision-making. The medical profession needs to be much more evidence-based in its practices, and utilize all available technology to get there as quickly as possible. Standardized EMR's, computers, and rigorous statistical analysis are key ingredients for reaching this goal.

For most of us, quality health care means personalized, evidence-based medicine that is affordable and accessible. The best evidence regarding efficacy, safety, convenience, and cost of treatment comes from rigorous statistical analysis on patients like you who have been through treatment. This kind evidence is far more reliable than flimflam stats and far more reliable than a doctor's opinion. But in order to benefit from the results of a rigorous statistical study, the patient has to be willing to give up a certain amount of pride in his personal uniqueness and allow himself to be viewed as a member of a cohort of similar patients – there is clear value in understanding the experience of the cohort.

Rigorous statistics supports not only personalized, evidence-based medicine, but also evidence-based public health policy. The latter is intended to serve society as a whole. True, sometimes it might deliver mandates that go against some people's personal preferences. There is nothing unusual in that – we've always have to give up a certain amount of personal freedom in order to reap the benefits of living in a society.

Today, many people in the US are opting for alternative medicine either as a substitute for or complement to conventional (Western) medicine. "CAM" is the acronym for complementary and alternative medicine. What's the difference between Western medicine and alternative medicine? In Western medicine, the mantra is: *In science we trust*. It has the ideal (still too often not achieved) of working like an applied science, with actions supported by scientific understanding of physics, chemistry, and biology, and by rigorous empirical evidence. Alternative medicine represents a more diverse and multi-cultural set of practices, often broken down by tradition, which seek to comfort and heal through body manipulation, "energy" manipulation, herbs, and tonics. Alternative medicine treatments are generally not well-supported by rigorous empirical evidence. Yet, most practitioners consider their work to be evidence-based, partly because some practices have a long history of use, and partly because each practice has its anecdotes of success.

People embrace alternative medicine for various reasons. Among them: a desire to be "healed naturally"; dissatisfaction with the limitations and side effects of Western medicine; and the often lower cost and easier access to alternative medicine. They may also point to the blunders of Western medicine as an argument that it should be altogether rejected.

Alternative medicine is a huge commercial industry – heavily promoted by flimflam stats. Alternative medicine is available on store shelves, at practitioner's offices, and now commonly at hospitals. A number of US states have written into law that health insurance must now cover certain types of alternative medical care.

Is alternative medicine effective? Is it more effective than Western medicine? Is one alternative medicine tradition better than another? How can we find out? Does it make sense for government to require that health insurance cover alternative medicine? Rigorous statistical analysis gives us an objective way of addressing these questions, in addition to questions about which Western treatments are best.

Most importantly, the patient who has a grasp of rigorous statistics is the patient who is best positioned to identify the most promising treatments for himself.

But I'm special

When it comes to finding the best treatment, some people believe that statistics about *any* group are irrelevant to their own particular situation – they see themselves as special.

I'm special, so special. I've got to have your attention. Give it to me now!

The Pretenders

But aren't we all special, so special? And we've got to have the doctor's attention now! Of course, if we're all so special, no amount of the doctor's attention is going to help. It's only when we allow ourselves to be viewed as not-so-special, viewed as similar to other patients who have been through treatment, that the idea of a best or most promising treatment has any real meaning, any possibility of being identified. After all, if nothing in medical experience resembles a case like ours, how is the doctor supposed to know how to treat us? Intuition? What?

When we go to the doctor's office, we are, in fact, quite used to being categorized – we fully expect to be measured, questioned, tested, and sized-up in all sorts of ways that allow the doctor to broadly categorize the kind of patient we are, and to register our symptoms. With millions of patients moving through the healthcare system every year, it stands to reason that there are probably hundreds, if not thousands, of historical patients who are similar to us in terms of gender, race, age, height, weight, blood pressure, family history, and all sorts of other particulars, who had the same health complaint we do and went through treatment. Rigorous statistical analysis on that cohort can yield invaluable information about our own prospects for success with this treatment or that.

But let's not forget that you *are* special. It's important to narrow the cohort of past patients to the right level. But if you narrow it to the point that no past patient is sufficiently similar to you, yes, treatment can still proceed – just recognize that something other than rigorous statistical evidence is being used to guide your treatment.

In the public interest

When deciding public policy on vaccination, health insurance, recreational drugs, personal freedoms, quarantine protocols, and standards for efficacy and safety, rigorous statistics are essential for making the best evidence-based decisions. Without it, politicians, drug manufacturers, device makers, and all sorts of other special interests will take charge, and we'll get nothing like best policy.

That said, rigorously-informed public health policy may be at odds with some people's personal preferences. That's to be expected. For example, some parents might prefer not to vaccinate their children against measles and polio – but that's in direct conflict with society's efforts to eradicate these diseases. Should society allow parents to withhold these vaccinations from their kids? Should society allow parents to withhold other vaccinations, such as for HPV? Should society allow parents to go the herbal or faith-healing route in tending to a sick child when Western medicine offers a treatment that is proven effective? And what about forced quarantining of a suspected case of Ebola? Such action can be viewed as a violation of personal freedom, but on the other hand, not taking that action risks spreading the disease. The individual may disagree with societal policies on smoking, drinking, and doing drugs, but if society is paying for the consequences of those choices, doesn't it have the right, indeed the obligation, to limit those choices?

Alternative medicine

>*Double, double toil and trouble;*
>*Fire burn and caldron bubble.*
>*Fillet of a fenny snake,*
>*In the caldron boil and bake;*
>*Eye of newt and toe of frog,*
>*Wool of bat and tongue of dog,*
>*Adder's fork and blind-worm's sting,*
>*Lizard's leg and howlet's wing,*
>*For a charm of powerful trouble,*
>*Like a hell-broth boil and bubble.*

>recipe from Shakespeare's Macbeth

Whatever it is that ails you, there's a medical practice that claims to have the cure. Sometimes it's Western medicine; sometimes it's alternative medicine. If it's alternative medicine, then you have many possibilities to choose from. You could go with one of the more ancient traditions like Ayurvedic medicine, Traditional Chinese Medicine, acupuncture, or cupping, which have been around for millennia. Or you could go with one of the more recent approaches like chiropractic, osteopathy, homeopathy, naturopathy, reflexology, Reiki, or Rolfing, which have been around for only a century or two. Most, if not all, of these practices – both the old and the new – are founded on elaborate theories and it usually takes a great deal of study to earn the accreditation necessary to practice.

Touching on some of the more ancient approaches: Ayurvedic medicine maintains that three humors control health and the practice seeks to balance these humors through medicinal preparations, physical manipulations, and chants; acupuncture is predicated on the flow of *qi* ("chi"), or "vital energy", along twelve meridians (pathways within the body), meticulously mapped by ancient practitioners; Traditional Chinese Medicine includes massage, acupuncture, herbalism, exercise, and diet, and is guided by cosmological philosophies such as Yin-Yang and The Five Phases; cupping therapy calls for special cups to be placed on the skin to create suction, which is claimed to help with a variety of ailments.

Touching on some of the more recent approaches: Reiki involves transfer of qi from the palms of the practitioner's hands to the patient's affected areas in order to encourage healing; Reflexology applies pressure to the patient's feet and hands to unblock qi from affected areas and promote healing; Rolfing kneads ligaments and tendons to impart suppleness, believed by practitioners to thwart a large variety of ills; Homeopathic remedies are prepared by repeatedly diluting a substance in alcohol or water, usually well beyond the point where even a single molecule of the original substance remains; Naturopathy employs homeopathy, herbalism, acupuncture, and diet; Osteopathy manipulates muscle and bone, with claims that this relieves a large variety of health conditions. Chiropractic manipulates the spine, under the belief that mechanical disorders of the spine impact general health via the nervous system. Traditional chiropractors perform these adjustments to unblock the flow of a supernatural energy called "innate intelligence" in order to cure what ails you.

And then there are the religious-based practices like faith healing and shamanism which seek divine or spiritual intervention for healing the body. Exorcism is still widely practiced today and serves those patients whose ills are caused by demonic possession.

Each of these practices and traditions has its avid supporters, expert practitioners, and mountains of anecdotes testifying to their efficacy. Each of these practices believes they are doing evidence-based medicine.

But this kind of evidence does not meet the standards of rigorous statistics. And when the latter standard is applied to the claims of alternative medicine, the treatments most often show themselves to be no better than sugar pills or contrived "sham" treatment. (For example, see "Research Casts Doubt on the Value of Acupuncture", *Scientific American*, Aug. 2016.)

Evidence-based medicine in Botswana

Our native guide knew all the plants in the area, their local names and medicinal uses: emetics, diuretics, aphrodisiacs, everything to address whatever concerns you coming or going. In the field, he pointed out a magnificent sausage tree (*Kigelia africana*), with mature sausage-shaped fruits up to a meter (40 in) in length.

He explained that in the village where he comes from, a small male member is a big problem – but that, fortunately, a solution is found in the sausage tree. The remedy for inadequate membership: Scratch the skin of an immature sausage fruit while it's still attached to the tree and rub some of its sap on your member. Then as the fruit increases in size, so too will your member. When enough is enough, you must return to the very same tree, locate the very same fruit, and cut it off the tree. Our guide claimed to know many people for whom the treatment worked like a charm. It worked very well for an uncle of his too, but, unfortunately, when it came time for him to quit the cure, he could not locate the tree.

As a result, his wife left him, and the uncle now lives alone.

At another village in Botswana, we were given a lecture and demonstration by the local witchdoctor. His hut was his apothecary, and the many shelves were lined with jars and cans of plant and animal stuff – stuff to be taken straight-up or accompanied by a ritual chant or dance. According to the villagers in attendance, his ministrations were very successful. One of the villagers acted out the symptoms of a women's ailment, an ailment that caused cramps and crazy behaviors. The witchdoctor-recommended the cure: Drink an infusion of elephant dung. According to the villagers, the treatment always worked. Now, isn't that evidence-based medicine?

So why do people believe in hokey practices? In some cases, it might be lack of exposure or access to other treatments. In other cases, it might be an attachment to cultural traditions. For the remainder, it might just be plain old gullibility and lack of critical thinking.

Conflicted medical practice

Medical training and practice today is enormously conflicted, at odds with itself. On the one hand, there's the call for rigorous evidence-based medicine. On the other hand, there's a widespread tilt toward complementary and alternative medicine (CAM), most of whose practices lack rigorous evidential support. Increasingly, medical schools are teaching CAM in the classroom, hospitals are offering CAM to their patients, and health insurance is being ordered to cover CAM.

This from the Wikipedia page on "Alternative Medicine": *In recent years, the number of med-schools offering courses in CAM has burgeoned to more than 50%. In 2008, more than 37.7% of American hospitals offered alternative therapies, up from 7.7% in 1999.*

How is it that CAM has been able to make such inroads into

institutions originally dedicated to Western medicine – medicine that aspires to be applied science? (See the "History" section of the Wikipedia page on "Alternative Medicine".)

Not surprisingly, it's about money. Public demand for CAM is gargantuan and growing, and everyone wants a piece of the action. In 2012, The National Center for Health Statistics reported that Americans spent over $30 billion on alternative medical products and services – that's $15 billion on practitioners, $13 billion on natural supplements, and $3 billion on self-care approaches. (See "Americans Spend $30 Billion a Year on Alternative Medicine", June 22, 2016, on nbcnews.com.) In 1990, 30% of Americans were using CAM. By 2013, 50% of Americans were using CAM. No wonder hospitals are offering services like acupuncture, cupping, Reiki, homeopathy, spiritual healing, and "detox programs". These are cash cows. (For a jaw-dropping account, see the article, "Medicine with a side of mysticism: Top hospitals promote unproven therapies", Mar. 7, 2017, on the website statnews.com)

However, in a rare pang of conscience or embarrassment, the clinical arm of UC Irvine abruptly dropped its newly-added homeopathy service after harsh criticism from the medical community concerned about patient health and well-being. (See "Facing criticism, UC Irvine scrubs homeopathy from its roster of offered treatments", *Los Angeles Times*, Sept. 25, 2017.)

Why is the public so inclined toward CAM? Various reasons: Some regard "natural" as safer and more effective than "synthetic" or surgical; some have a blanket distrust of the medical establishment; some are frustrated by the limitations and side effects they've experienced with Western medicine; some cite a lack of good communication with their Western-style doctors; and some point to the blunders of Western medicine.

Another part of the explanation lies in the public's confusion over what constitutes Western medicine versus alternative medicine. Some recommendations that CAM practitioners would have you believe are "alternative" are in fact well-researched and fully-recognized by Western medicine as promoting health. This includes attention to diet, exercise, and stress reduction. To the extent that Western medicine acknowledges the importance of these items, they should not be considered "alternative". Similarly, alternative medicine does not have a lock on herbs, as we'll see later.

Another factor that has contributed to the rise of CAM is political influence. In the early 1990's, Sen. Tom Harkin, at the prodding of influential constituents, began promoting alternative medicine and allocating large sums of federal money to test and validate alternative treatments. Later, in 1994, Sen. Harkin and Sen. Orrin Hatch introduced legislation that decreased the FDA's authority to inform consumers about misleading claims on products sold as natural supplements. As a result, few consumers are aware that most of the claims made by supplement manufacturers are not supported by rigorous evidence.

To date, no significant findings have been made in favor of alternative medicine. From 1999 to 2009, the federal government spent over $2.5 billion tax dollars on randomized controlled trials through the Office of Alternative Medicine (OAM), which later became the National Center for Complementary and Alternative Medicine (NCCAM), and came up empty-handed: Echinacea for colds, Ginkgo biloba for memory, glucosamine and chondroitin for arthritis, black cohosh for menopausal hot flashes, saw palmetto for prostate problems, shark cartilage for cancer – all these and others proved no better than dummy pills. (See "$2.5 billion spent, no alternative cures found", June 10, 2009, on nbcnews.com.)

Yet, many believers will never be convinced that the bulk of CAM practices and claims are unsubstantiated. Hope, fear, desperation, and a yearning to be "healed naturally" will continue to drive strong demand for CAM products and services.

All said, there is one herb in the cabinet of alternative medicine that has definitely not received enough scientific study – and that's marijuana. Numerous small studies and much anecdotal evidence indicate that cannabis, smoked, vaporized, or distilled into a skin ointment (involving CBD oil and THC) is very helpful for combatting neuropathic pain, nausea, and anxiety in patients undergoing chemotherapy. (See for example, the page "Marijuana and Cancer" on the website of the American Cancer Society.) There is anecdotal evidence that in some patients, marijuana-based skin ointment is more effective at relieving neuropathic pain than opioid drugs, while being less addictive and producing fewer side effects. There is anecdotal evidence that in some patients, marijuana-based extract (involving CBD oil and THC) is more effective at relieving post-operative pain than opioid drugs, while being less addictive and producing fewer side effects. It is very unfortunate that the US federal government does not support research into the medical potential of the marijuana plant.

Blunders in Western medicine

Contemporary Western medicine, which originated in twentieth century Europe and the US, is not directed by a single, unifying principle that guides all diagnosis and treatment. There are no notions of universal energy fields, energy pathways, innate intelligence, humors, or chakras that somehow get out of whack and need their proper balance or flow restored. Instead, Western medicine developed from a hodge-podge of ideas inspired by contemporary science (physics, chemistry, and biology), and like science, the ideal seeks rigorous empirical support for its theories and practices.

Following this paradigm, Western medicine has demonstrated many remarkable successes. But it has also made its share of blunders, some of which we'll see in a moment. Some proponents of alternative medicine point to the blunders of Western medicine as grounds to dismiss the whole tradition. That makes no sense. Progress in any scientific field involves making mistakes and learning from those mistakes. The field of engineering has made numerous blunders in the course of history – but given its many accomplishments, no one suggests tossing the discipline out the window. Western medicine has been wildly successful in treating and preventing many diseases and conditions. When it makes mistakes, at least there is a mechanism for recognizing those mistakes and refining the body of accepted knowledge and practice accordingly. Of course, it is helpful to discover those mistakes as soon as possible.

Here are some examples over the last forty years where Western medicine got it wrong:

- Prior to the 1980's, gastroenterologists took the psychological state of the patient as the leading cause of stomach ulcers. Today, they look instead for the presence of the bacterium *Helicobactor pylori*.

- The prescription drug 'Fen-Phen" (for appetite suppression and weight loss) hit the market in the early 1990s and gained widespread usage. Though the FDA had previously approved the constituent drugs, fenfluramine and phentermine, for separate use, the agency never approved them for use in combination – and that's where the problem arose – in their combination. By 1997, high rates of severe cardiac injury were being reported, and the drug was pulled from the market shortly thereafter.

  Similarly, the drugs, Avandia (for diabetes), Vioxx (for arthritis pain), and Celebrex (for arthritis pain), were all cleared as safe and effective by the FDA in the late 1990's, but post-market surveillance showed major safety problems.

- The PSA test was approved by the FDA in 1994 for use as a screening tool in diagnosing prostate cancer. But in 2009, two major studies, both involving tens of thousands of men without risk factors, concluded that the survivorship of men who tested positive and were then biopsied, diagnosed, and treated, was no greater than that of a control population who did not undergo the test. (See the article, "The Great Prostate Debate: Does Screening Save Lives?", *Scientific American*, Feb. 2012. See also, "Marc Garnick Answers 6 Key Questions about Prostate Cancer" in the same issue.) Beginning in 2011, the USPSTF now recommends against the PSA test for healthy men without risk factors, stating that the potential benefit does not outweigh the risks of harm.

- For women diagnosed with ductile carcinoma in situ (DCIS), also known as Stage 0 breast cancer, the standard treatment for decades has been surgery (mastectomy or lumpectomy), followed by radiation and chemo. Since 2009, strong evidence has emerged that most of these cancers are slow-growing and will not threaten life – implying that aggressive treatment has for the most part been over-treatment. The new thinking is that active surveillance and drug therapy is the best way to address a diagnosis of DCIS. (See "Why Doctors are Rethinking Breast-Cancer Treatment", *Time*, Oct. 1, 2015.)

- For decades, Hormone Replacement Therapy (HRT) was widely prescribed for relief from the symptoms of menopause. But in 2002, an extensive Women's Health Initiative study determined that HRT was linked to significantly increased rates of breast cancer, coronary heart disease, and stroke. No longer is HRT recommended as a blanket therapy for post-menopausal women.

- Since the late 1980s, stent insertion to unclog coronary arteries has been one of the most common heart surgeries. But a landmark study published in the New England Journal of Medicine in 2007 concluded that (quote): *as an initial management strategy in patients with stable coronary artery disease, [stent insertion] does not reduce the risk of death, myocardial infarction, or other major cardiovascular events when added to optimal medical therapy.* Ten years later, the procedure is still widely used, without evidence to justify it. (See "Thousands of heart patients get stents that may do more harm than good", *Vox*, Nov. 6, 2017, which cites a major study that appeared subsequently in *The Lancet*, Jan. 2018. See also, "Heart stents are useless for most stable patients. They're still widely used.", *New York Times*, Feb. 12, 2018.)

- Since the 1970's, many large class action lawsuits have been filed on behalf of patients who were harmed by implanted devices. These devices include: the Dalkon Shield, silicone breast implants, vaginal meshes, and various designs of hip prostheses. Though the Dalkon Shield was introduced before the FDA had authority to regulate devices, the other implants were introduced after.

- There is still a high rate of preventable medical errors leading to adverse drug reactions in patients: Among the sources of error: wrong drug prescribed; wrong dosage or duration prescribed; bad interaction between drugs.

Hope and desperation

We are a suggestible species. We want to believe in something, particularly when things are not going well, particularly when we are suffering and in pain. We want to believe in something that will lead to a long and healthy life. This sets us up as the perfect mark for those making big promises, pushing products and services of questionable benefit. The pitch usually involves flimflam stats. Mostly what these parties are selling, and mostly what alternative medicine sells, is artfully-packaged, artfully-delivered, positive suggestion – which usually equates to **placebo**. (For us, a placebo is any health intervention that lacks rigorous statistical evidence for efficacy beyond the "do nothing" treatment.) For some conditions, mere positive suggestion does appear to be more effective than doing nothing – but this has only been demonstrated in relation to stress, hypertension, depression, and certain kinds of pain. There is no convincing evidence that positive suggestion alone is effective in treating cancer, diabetes, arthritis, infection, kidney stones, and many other serious conditions and diseases.

Although alternative medicine may benefit some, it's use is not always without risk. A true believer might be lulled into thinking that his condition has been adequately addressed, when in fact, a serious underlying biological cause remains hidden and unaddressed. In going the alternative route, the believer may be postponing or forgoing a Western-style treatment that is known to be highly effective, possibly missing a crucial window of opportunity, which could end up shortening life or impacting quality of life.

Should it be mandated that health insurance cover alternative medicine? Is alternative medicine cost effective? On the one hand, alternative medicine in the US is often cheaper and more accessible than Western treatment. On the other hand, in pursuing alternative treatment for a serious condition, the patient might miss the window of opportunity for easy and effective Western treatment. If the patient's condition worsens, and the patient finally decides to go the Western route, heroic measures may be required at great expense. This would not be cost effective.

Comparing medical traditions

Every medical tradition boasts its successes and downplays its failures. So, how do we choose which one to stake our health and lives on?

Just as rigorous statistics can be used to compare medications, procedures, doctors, and hospitals, it can also be used to compare treatments from different medical traditions – again, by looking at historical patient outcomes, and assessing treatment efficacy, safety, convenience, and cost.

Of course, the alternative traditions will argue with one another and with the Western tradition about what characterizes an ailment, its symptoms, and successful treatment. Some will insist on considering unobservables, intangibles, and unmeasurables – disingenuous ruses to confuse and obfuscate. So getting to the point where non-controversial comparisons can be made isn't easy. But in the interest of doing so, it is crucial that the competing traditions agree on a description of the ailment and on the definition of successful treatment.

Suppose, for example, that we wish to compare the efficacy of acupuncture against Western treatment for what the latter would call "frozen shoulder". We first have to ask if acupuncture recognizes the symptoms of frozen shoulder as a treatable condition, regardless of what name they give to this batch of symptoms. Then we have to get agreement from both traditions as to what constitutes a cure or improvement. With these agreements, a non-controversial statistical comparison of efficacy is possible.

But even within the same tradition, getting agreement on diagnosis and the definition of successful treatment is not always easy. For example, in the Western tradition, should aggressive treatment of a tumor that is not usually life-threatening be considered a successful treatment? Not all doctors agree on the answer. A similar question arises when talking about cardiac oblation for the control of atrial fibrillation – what are the criteria of a successful treatment? When talking about mental health disorders: Is it a disorder? Does it meet the threshold? Is it treatable? What is the definition of successful treatment? These questions are often controversial. But, again, if we want to be able to compare treatments, there first has to be agreement on definitions.

When comparing two traditions as a whole, if the treatments of one, across a variety of ailments, are statistically superior to the other, then clearly it makes sense to favor the tradition with the statistical advantage.

Whether within tradition or across traditions, it might be that two treatments show similar efficacy and safety. That motivates further comparison by invasiveness, burden to patient, and cost to the healthcare system. An interesting example is the set of Western options for treating clubfoot in children. Until recently, the prevailing treatment involved a significant surgery to lengthen muscles and tendons. This treatment has demonstrated a high rate of good outcomes. However, that technique is now being replaced by the "Ponseti method", a non-surgical or minimally-surgical technique developed in the 1950's that relies almost entirely on foot manipulation and serial casting. Another non-surgical technique involves the use of Botox. (See the article on "clubfoot" in Wikipedia. See also the article, "This simple correction for clubfoot is a life changer for kids in India", *PBS NewsHour*, July 3, 2017.)

Here's another example of two treatments in Western medicine, both widely used, where one is much less invasive than the other: lumpectomy versus mastectomy for localized breast cancer. Both methods offer similar survival rates according to the website breastcancer.org (see "Mastectomy vs. Lumpectomy").

If it works, it works

Science places a high value on theoretical understanding, on logical deductions from well-stated premises that make accurate predictions about the world. Predictive theories are not only intellectually satisfying, but they often give rise to powerful applications and further insights down the road. The scientific theories developed in physics, chemistry, and biology, have proven astonishingly fruitful, enabling all the engineering marvels around us and providing deep insights into the workings of the human body.

Alternative medicine is often criticized for being hokey and implausible in its explanations that drive treatment. The explanations are typically at odds with scientific theory and scientific understanding of how the world works. Science has no explanation for how magnetic fields, rock crystals, and homeopathic liquids can possibly heal the body. But implausible explanation or lack of explanation does not mean that a treatment is ineffective. A treatment's efficacy should be determined by the quality of its collective outcomes, independent of underlying theory. (However, regrading safety, it might be prudent to entertain theoretical arguments against the safety of a treatment.) Such an approach is "tradition-agnostic" – it doesn't care if the treatment comes from Western medicine or alternative medicine.

In fact, Western medicine – which values scientific explanation for its practices – is replete with treatments that proved effective long before their mechanisms of action were understood. In some cases, those mechanisms are still not understood even today. But if it works, it works! Here are some examples:

- The potent beneficial properties of certain plants were known for hundreds, even thousands, of years before twentieth-century science was able to understand some of the underlying biochemistry: willow bark (contains salicylic acid, "aspirin", to treat pain, fever, and inflammation); cinchona bark (contains quinine, an anti-malarial); autumn crocus (contains colchicine to treat gout); belladonna (contains atropine and hyoscine to treat intestinal cramping); foxglove (contains digitalin to control heart rate); opium poppy (contains morphine and codeine, powerful pain-killers); and Pacific yew bark (contains paclitaxel, an important chemotherapy drug for cancer). Western medicine recognizes the effectiveness of peppermint oil (for symptoms of irritable bowel syndrome) and green tea (for treating genital warts and high cholesterol). Hence, it cannot be said that Western medicine ignores herbs. But its standard for acceptance is much higher than in alternative medicine.

- Since antiquity it was known that eating liver could cure night blindness (now known to be caused by vitamin A deficiency). The curative effects of lemons and limes on scurvy (now known to be caused by vitamin C deficiency) were known at least as far back as the fifteenth century. The curative effect of cod liver oil on rickets (a result of vitamin D deficiency) was recognized in the later 1800's. All these treatments were observed to be effective well before twentieth century scientific understanding of vitamin biochemistry.

- Alexander Fleming first isolated the chemical penicillin from the *Penicillium* mold in 1928. He and scientists before him observed that *Penicillium* could destroy bacteria in a Petri dish. Penicillin was first mass produced as an antibiotic beginning in 1945, but its mechanism of action was not understood until later. Today, there is considerable dispute over the means by which a host of newer antibiotics suppress and destroy bacteria.

- The first recorded use of inoculation took place in China in the fifteenth century. To confer protection against smallpox, dried, powdered, smallpox scabs were blown into the nostrils of the recipient. At the time, people knew nothing of viruses, bacteria, antibodies, or white blood cells. The germ theory of disease was first proposed by Girolamo Fracastoro in 1546 and rejected for centuries. By the mid-1800's, the germ theory of disease was taking hold, but the microscopic workings of the immune system were still a complete mystery. And yet, between 1870 and 1880, Jean-Joseph-Henri Toussaint, Emil Roux, and Louis Pasteur successfully created vaccines for anthrax and rabies.

- Without knowledge of the underlying biochemistry, the 1950's saw the introduction of chlorpromazine (Thorozine) for psychoses and lithium carbonate for mania, beginning a revolution in psychopharmacology. To this day, we still do not understand how either drug works.

- Prozac, first marketed in 1986, is an antidepressant in the class of selective serotonin reuptake inhibitors. Yet much about its biochemical action is still not understood.

- Acetaminophen (the active ingredient in Tylenol), discovered in 1887, has been available as a non-prescription pain reliever since 1960. Its mechanism of action is still unknown.

- The mechanism of action behind general anesthesia remains a complete mystery to this day.

- Viagra was first marketed in 1998. The active ingredient was initially developed to treat angina and hypertension. It didn't pan out for angina, but showed surprising success in treating erectile dysfunction.

- Thalidomide was first marketed in 1957 for insomnia and

morning sickness in pregnant women. Shortly after, it was linked to a high rate of severe birth defects and pulled from the market. Later, it was discovered to be an effective drug in treating leprosy, and was FDA-approved it for that in 1998.

A revolution in the way medical decisions are made

You get what you pay for – or maybe not – at least not with medical care in the US. And whatever it is that we are paying for, we can't afford it.

Patients need rigorous, personalized, evidence-based answers to the following sorts of questions: What are the odds this treatment will help me? How well do we know those odds? Similarly, what are the odds this treatment will harm me? How well do we know those odds? How do the numbers for this treatment compare with those of that treatment?

Presently, the healthcare system is not answering these questions for patients. A revolution is needed in the way medical decisions are made – a revolution based on the idea that identifying best treatment options for the current patient is possible only with access to rigorous statistics on similar patients who have been through treatment. This is the only way to get personalized, objective information about treatment performance, where the reliability of that information, as a predictor of future performance, can itself be quantified in a meaningful way through confidence intervals. Such a strategy lets historical patient data do all the talking, instead of subjective and corruptible "expert opinion" and any sort of flimflam stats. The only subjectivity that should enter into a medical decision is that of the patient expressing his own personal preferences.

The paradigm of rigorous statistics enables comparisons of drugs, procedures, doctors, hospitals, and even medical traditions. When combined with electronic medical records, the paradigm enables patients to understand which treatments are most likely to be beneficial. This understanding will change in time as more medical records enter the system and new treatments come into existence. The paradigm will curtail overtreatment – procedures and prescriptions that do not serve patients well and lard the cost of healthcare.

Who will spearhead the revolution? – not Big Pharma; not device makers; not hospital CEO's; and not doctors. They're happy with the way things are. They don't want any change that could impact the bottom line. Doctors don't want their authority, prestige, knowledge, and judgement challenged. They don't want to be burdened with more things to study, like rigorous statistics. And they don't want to be pressured to adjust their practices based on what the statistics indicate. In the article, "The birth of a new American aristocracy", *The Atlantic*, June 2018, author Matthew Stewart says that many economists liken US physician's organizations to a cartel, using their power to control pricing and availability. He levels the same criticism against dentistry and the pharmaceutical industry. But this state of affairs does not exist in other industrialized nations.

So others have to spearhead the revolution. This includes patients who demand rigorous statistical evidence as a prerequisite to treatment.

The ingredients needed for the revolution are here today: computing power; statistical algorithms; efficient databases; and large repositories of electronic medical records that are becoming increasingly standardized. The issues of data integrity, privacy, and security are being tackled.

Recently, some companies in the health care analytics industry have begun to offer platforms that support data analysis on user-selected cohorts of historical patients. We are not aware if these services are available directly to patients, nor are we aware of the exact capabilities and limitations of these systems, the quality of their analyses and reports, and the degree to which they are being used by the medical profession.

In the revolution, patients have direct access to this kind of service. The patient fills out an electronic questionnaire that asks for medical history and symptoms, and allows for treatment preferences to be entered. Based on answers to the questionnaire, the system then taps into a huge database of anonymous standardized EMR's and identifies patients similar to the current patient who have been through treatment. It analyzes these patients and reports back rigorous statistics on treatment performance: the observed rates of benefits and harms associated with each treatment, and their confidence intervals. The report further includes: the filters used to identify patients similar to the current patient; the filters used to limit the kinds of treatments considered (e.g., non-surgical), and the filters used to limit what is reported (e.g., suppress information on treatments that have small sample sizes). The patient will be able to adjust these filters to satisfy his own requirements.

The level of knowledge required to understand such a report is surprisingly modest and was covered in Chapters 7 through 10. But not every patient has the time or interest to get that understanding. These patients will need a new kind of advisor, one capable of explaining how the patient uses such a report to evaluate and compare treatments, and why the methodology is worthy of trust. This new medical professional does not have to have a medical degree or know how to administer medical procedures or treatments, but will have to know the basics of statistical analysis and have good teaching and inter-personal skills. In fact, it is our feeling that this professional *should not* have a medical degree, so as to avoid any intrinsic bias favoring one treatment approach over another that might arise from med school training or an opportunity for financial gain. Best treatment can only be identified through statistical evidence, patient understanding of that evidence, and patient preferences.

We might call such a practitioner a "medical decision advisor", with the acronym MDA.

The need for a massive change in the way health care is delivered in the US is urgent. Let's get on with it.

Meanwhile, stay well!

Jerome Malitz and Seth Malitz

Where's the Bibliography?

If you are looking for a traditional bibliography, you won't find it here. In the past, a big fat bibliography was a must for serious works of non-fiction. Here we're doing it differently for several reasons:

First of all, most of our sources are fully cited within the body of the text. So in this sense, the whole book is itself a bibliography.

Secondly, those citations represent sources that were actually consulted – we do not wish to lard a bibliography with sources that were not consulted.

Thirdly, we used very few books. These include some textbooks that we tortured students with during our teaching days. If we were to teach probability and statistics again to a senior-level college audience with students from a wide variety of disciplines, we would use the present book as our primary text.

So, for these reasons, we leave you unencumbered by a traditional bibliography.

Index

(*a*, *c*)-good, 133
ABCDE method (melanoma screening), 38, 179
absolute risk
 increase (ARI), 187
 reduction (ARR), 186
accuracy
 absolute, 132
 relative, 132
Arrow's Paradox, 192
average, 119
bar chart, 96
Bayes' Theorem, 114, 116
bell curve, 91
bias, forms of, 148
Binomial distribution, 127
 fractional, 127
Central Limit Theorem (CLT), 131
choose operation, 86
concentration of probability about the mean, 128
confidence, 132
confidence interval, 133
control group, 184
covariance matrix, 126
cutoff
 boundary, 179
 curve, 179
 value, 177
data dredging, 152
decision tree, 193
disease risk curve, 177
disease risk surface, 180
electronic medical record (EMR), 29
event, 85
events
 correlation between, 110
 dependent, 109

disjoint, 105, 109
 independent, 109
 operations on, 104, 105
exact method, 134, 135, 137
expected value, 119
experimental group, 184
extrapolation, 173
false negative, 105
 probability, 107
 rate, 107
false positive, 105
 probability, 107
 rate, 107
flimflam stats, 217
gold standard test, 111
histogram. *See* probability histogram
histogram of sample means, 128
hypothesis testing, statistical, 137
interpolation, 173
lab developed test (LDT), 115
Law of Large Numbers, 132
Law of Truly Large Numbers, 153
Maximum Likelihood Estimation, 170
mean, 119
 in higher dimensions, 126
 of binary experiment, 120
 of binary population, 120
 of probability curve, 124
median, 121
melanoma. *See* ABCDE method
meta-analysis (study), 145
mode, 121
natural language processing, 141, 225
negative prediction value, 107
Normal distribution curve, 91,

    124
    Standard, 125
number needed to
    harm (NNH), 187
    screen (NNS), 187
    treat (NNT), 187
off-label drug use (OLDU), 56
pie chart, 95
placebo, 248
population, 85
positive prediction value, 107
predicate device, 59
Pre-Market Notification 510(k), 59
prevalence, 103
probability
    by counting, 85
    conditional, 106
    distribution, 101
    distribution curve, 92
    histogram, 94
    Kolmogorov axioms, 100
    measure, 100
    of an event, 85
    posterior, 116
    prior, 116
    theory, 101
regression
    analysis, 158
    best-fit model, 164
    curve fit, 159
    factor, 158
    factor reduction, 171
    goodness-of-fit, 164
    input variable, 158

    least squares method, 164
    linear, 165
    mean squared error, 165
    model, 159
    output variable, 158
    over-fit, 166
    signal and noise, 159
    surface fit, 159
    under-fit, 166
    vertical residual, 164
relative risk
    increase (RRI), 187
    reduction (RRR), 186
reproducibility, statistical, 216
rigorous statistics, 216
sample size approximation
    formula, 131, 134
sensitivity (of test), 107
Simpson's Paradox, 149
specificity (of test), 107
standard deviation, 122
structured data, 141
success rate (of treatment), 188
total error probability, 107
total weighted error, 107
Turing machine, 31
unstructured data, 141
vaccine effectiveness, 185
variance, 122
    in higher dimensions, 126
    of binary experiment, 123
    of binary population, 123
    of probability curve, 124
Venn diagram, 104

ABOUT THE AUTHORS

The authors, father and son, are Ph.D. mathematicians.

Jerome Malitz received his doctorate from the University of California at Berkeley in 1966, and is now Prof. Emeritus at the University of Colorado, having taught there for thirty years.

Seth Malitz received his doctorate from MIT in 1988, and served on the faculty at UMASS Amherst until 1992. Since 2005, he has been a research and development scientist at GeoEye and DigitalGlobe.

OTHER BOOKS BY THE AUTHORS

Introduction to Mathematical Logic, Jerome Malitz, 1979.

Personal Landscapes, Jerome Malitz, 1989.

Rocky Mountain National Park Dayhiker's Guide, Jerome Malitz, 1993.

Plants for the Future: A Gardener's Wishbook, Jerome Malitz, 1996.

Reflecting Nature: Garden Design from Wild Landscapes, Jerome Malitz and Seth Malitz, 1998.

Interior Landscapes, Horticulture and Design, Jerome Malitz and Seth Malitz, 2002.

Arches National Park Dayhiker's Guide, Jerome Malitz and Susan Malitz, 2005.

Acadia National Park Dayhiker's Guide, Jerome Malitz and Susan Malitz, 2007.

Gullible Us, Jerome Malitz, 2011.

Commode Contemplations, Jerome Malitz, 2017.

Commode Contemplations 2nd MVT, Jerome Malitz, 2018.

www.ingramcontent.com/pod-product-compliance
Lightning Source LLC
Chambersburg PA
CBHW071631220526
45469CB00002B/574